INTERMITTENT FASTING FOR WOMEN OVER 50

THE SCIENCE-BACKED 3-STEP GUIDE TO LOSE WEIGHT, BOOST ENERGY AND LONGEVITY, ALL WITHOUT COUNTING CALORIES!

KENDALL PETERS

D1736273

CONTENTS

INTRODUCTION

"Eliminate the mindset of can't - because you can do anything"

— TONY HORTON

Two years ago I was around at a friend's house, and unusually for her she was a bit down. Normally the life and soul of the party, that day Jane said she was finding it a bit difficult to motivate herself to get some boring admin done, that she said had been hanging over her for days, but didn't elaborate further. Jane is one of those people who will only tell you something when she's ready. So I waited. And over the course of the afternoon it slowly came out...

"I know I should expect it now I'm in my fifties, because I know metabolism slows down, but I don't like the way I look any more, and I don't feel there is anything I can do about it. Lord knows I've tried. I eat healthily, I walk to and from school every day (she's a teacher), I take a spin class when I can, and yet, over the last few years, I just feel that clothes are getting tighter, my body's getting saggier, and I hate that I don't seem to be able to change that. I've tried several diets, but they don't work. And the menopause isn't helping! Hot flushes, awake half the night, being tired all of the time. And don't get me started on the brain fog…I've got my parents to look after, and I know my kids are growing up, and will fly the nest soon, but I still want to be a role model to them, to show them that age is a number, and that you can be fit and healthy at any age, but at the moment, I feel I'm failing in that department. What am I going to do?"

There was clearly a lot to unpack, but rather than ask her about each point, I asked her what she was looking for, what her dream end-game looked like. After thinking about it for a few seconds, she said,

"I just want some 'zip' back. I don't want to feel tired all the time, I want to feel in control of my body, and oh, I want to lose weight that I can keep off without dieting constantly. I didn't look bad before I had kids if you remember. "

I did remember. When she was younger she definitely didn't lack for attention! She still looks great, but I felt she didn't want to hear it at that moment.

What I did tell her was that she wasn't failing, just struggling. It's something I tell myself whenever I feel things are going badly. You're not failing, just struggling.

I reminded her that she was in one of the hardest stages in life, the 'sandwich-generation', when you often have to look after your parents as well as your children, often while trying to hold down a demanding job, probably keeping the home looking nice and dealing with first-world life admin. On top of that, she was right, the menopause definitely wasn't helping, with sleep-deprivation making everything feel so much worse. And on top of all *that*, women tend to put others first, always thinking about what their kids need, what their parents need, what their partner needs, and rarely about what they themselves need. There's a reason why in airplane safety briefings they tell you to put a mask on your-self first before helping others, but sometimes women don't think like that.

I also told her that I had the answers to many of her issues. I told her I could show her how to lose weight without dieting and counting calories, and that the same process would boost her energy by making her body more insulin-sensitive (much more on this later). And by losing weight and having more energy, she would become much more confident about her body and in a much better place to tackle life, both good and bad. That she could be healthy for the rest of her life, and maybe even extend it!

"Bull****" she said. " How?"

So over the next couple of hours I told her how I've been intermittent fasting off and on for the last fifteen years, in all of its various forms. I told her how it works, why it works, the different ways to do it, how not to do it, the physical benefits it gives, and the effectiveness, simplicity and flexibility with which it can be fitted into your lifestyle. I told her about the scientific papers I had read on the subject. And all the anecdotal evidence on social media from countless people who all said it worked for them.

She said, "How come I didn't know you did this?" I repeated the effectiveness, simplicity and flexibility part. One of the many great things about intermittent fasting is that it doesn't have to affect anyone else as it is so easily adapted.

And I showed her that it works. I borrowed her laptop, got YouTube up, and typed in 'intermittent fasting' into the search bar (do this yourself now so you can see what I showed Jane). I didn't play her the videos, but I showed her the comments underneath a few of the videos, all from people who rave about fasting, telling how many pounds they have lost. I then did the same in Reddit.com and Quora.com, with the same results. Thousands and thousands of people like you and me, all saying they have lost weight by intermittent fasting.

She said, "You should write a book about this." I told her that books on the subject existed already, and that I would buy one for her.

And I did. In fact, I bought about five, all on Amazon. The ones with the most reviews and the highest rankings. I read them all, cover to cover, looking for the best one to hand over to Jane. And I was shocked.

There were six areas that made me not recommend any of them to Jane:

- The amount of typos and poor grammar in a lot of them instantly made me distrust the people who wrote them. To see what I mean, go to the reviews and see how many of the 3, 2 and 1-star reviews mention typos.
- Lots of options were given for different fasting plans, but little direction was given to help the reader decide which was best for them. It was often a case of 'here are the choices, you decide'
- Many of them also didn't have many, or even any, references to the science behind their claims, which sometimes made me doubt the claim made
- Intermittent fasting was being touted as a cure-all for the menopause. Fasting will definitely help with a lot of symptoms, but it won't replace estrogen
- The books targeted women over 50 from a marketing perspective, but when it came to outlining reasons why women over 50 should practice IF, the reasons given were generic to both genders and all age groups

- The recipes were often for things that weren't very appealing, or had confusing instructions. Again this is backed up by others in their 1,2 and 3-star reviews

So I decided to take Jane's advice and write a book about it, in which I corrected the issues found in other books, and outlined a simple 3-step guide to arm the reader with all the knowledge needed to get her on the right fasting path straight away.

And I can show you all this too. After reading this book, you will:

- Learn how to lose weight easily, without the suffering that comes with diets
- Discover all you need to know about intermittent fasting and the best way to do it
- Have a tool you can use for the rest of your life to keep you at a healthy weight
- Gain much more energy to deal with all that life throws at you
- Be more confident in yourself
- And crucially, reduce your risk from the main killers of heart disease, strokes, cancer, diabetes, dementia and obesity considerably

As a result, your quality of life will increase because you will be in a lot better place both physically and mentally. Maybe that's becoming more physically active, playing with grandkids more, doing more traveling, or being more focused while at work. The list is endless. And all it takes is to read this book and start your own journey.

I'm going to show you, in 3 simple steps, how to 1) pick the best method of intermittent fasting for you to start with, 2) how to decide what you're going to eat (with no calorie-counting), and 3) how to start off with the best possible chance of success.

Before we start on that journey, we're going to dive into what intermittent fasting is (and isn't), the different types, and the massive health benefits that you'll get by doing it, most of which don't come via dieting. And I'm also going to show you, scientifically, why it *will* work for you.

We'll also discuss why intermittent fasting is particularly beneficial for women over 50, as well as how fasting and exercise can co-exist.

By the time you've finished the book I honestly believe that you will be itching to get started, and wishing you had learnt about it years ago. But it's never too late!

A bit about me. I am Kendall Peters, a personal trainer and nutritional advisor. My work focuses on fitness, health, and nutrition for the over 50s, catering to both men and women. I have worked with people at every stage of adulthood, but the majority of my current clients are over 50. As a trainer and adviser also in my 50s, I have found out, from my 25 years of experience, that fitness and nutrition advice for older adults is more difficult to find, and I have come to understand that many don't understand how their needs have changed as they've gotten older. This book guides women over 50 on how to turn back the clock, regain their youth, and be confident in themselves with IF. I want you to know that you are not alone and I have been able to help countless people within this age bracket, in presenting a better life through the adoption of a better nutritional and healthier lifestyle. The process is not tedious, it just needs a small amount of discipline and decision-infused routines, to make a lasting change in your life.

Because the aim of this book is to change your life. It's a lofty aim, but the benefits of being able to know how to control your own weight and increase your energy levels will have a massive knock-on effect on all parts of your life, and it can all be done with just small changes to your daily routine. It doesn't necessarily mean you need to eat less, although that will probably end up happening, it just means that you need to eat between certain times of the day, but we'll go through all this and more. We'll discuss what IF is, what the science behind it is, what its benefits are, the different types of IF, the best one to start with, and the pitfalls to avoid. We'll discuss whether you need to change your current diet (spoiler alert, the answer is 'no' unless you eat cream cakes or fast food all day) and how to fit it into your current daily routine. We'll also discuss exercise, and the myths around IF. Finally I've put some recipes at the end along with a couple of meal plans if you decide that healthier meals might be a route for you.

So all the questions that may be running through your mind, like *'What happens when I'm hungry?' 'Can I exercise?' 'Can I have sweeteners in my coffee?' 'What times of the day should I be doing this?'* etc will all be answered in the following pages.

And now the easy bit. The 3 steps talked about in the title are two decisions and one action.

The 3 steps are to

1. Decide which IF type is the best to get started with
2. Decide whether to eat the way you do now or whether healthier alternatives are an option
3. Start your fasting journey, making sure you set yourself up to succeed

At the end of this book, you will have gained insight, knowledge, and know-how on using this powerful tool, intermittent fasting, to better your health, lose weight, and most importantly, help achieve your desired lifestyle.

Let's get started!

1

WHY INTERMITTENT FASTING
WILL WORK FOR YOU

In this chapter we'll discuss what intermittent fasting is, the different ways to fast, the science behind why fasting works, and the benefits you will gain from doing it. In particular we'll discuss the two main reasons why IF works.

WHAT INTERMITTENT FASTING IS

Let's quickly cover the basics. Intermittent fasting is a way of eating that involves changing regularly between periods of eating and fasting, i.e deliberately not eating. The fasting window may be measured in hours or days, and includes the time when you are asleep. When the fasting period is measured in hours, IF is also known as time-restricted eating. When fasting lasts for 24 hours or more, it tends to be called a specific name, such as 5:2, or OMAD (One Meal A

Day). We will go into the main types in detail in Chapter Three.

WHAT INTERMITTENT FASTING IS NOT

IF is not a diet. I repeat, IF is not a diet. The main characteristic of diets is the caloric restriction that is imposed to achieve the desired result. Most diets usually restrict a few things from your normal diet, which means you end up hungry nearly all the time.

This is the selling point of intermittent fasting. Rather than telling you *what* to eat, it tells you *when* to eat, so you can still, if you want, continue to eat what you do currently, only instead of eating it throughout your waking hours, you will restrict that intake to a certain number of hours a day. How many hours a day is discussed in Chapter Three.

One of the advantages of IF is the flexibility of the plan. You can use it as little or as much as you want. Some people mix and match it throughout the year, others mix and match the types of IF they do. All the different methods have been proven to be effective, but Chapter Three suggests the best one to start with.

Below is a brief introduction into the main types of fasting, but they are covered in more detail later on.

TIME-RESTRICTED EATING (TRE)

There are many time windows available in this type of IF. This type of fasting can easily be incorporated into your daily life. The rule of thumb is that you restrict eating into a 4-11-hour window while you fast for the remaining 13-20 hours. A lot of people adjust their fasting according to their schedules. Below are some of the most popular variations of time-restricted eating.

16:8

People usually eat 2-3 meals within 8 hours and fast in the remaining 16 hours. Remember, the time asleep counts as part of the fasting window. The longer you can sleep, the easier it is to fast! A typical day would involve having your first meal at around midday, which could be breakfast or lunch, and finishing eating dinner at 8pm, drinking only water or black tea/coffee in between those hours.

20:4

The 20:4 is a time-restrictive eating type based on 20 hours of fasting and 4 hours of eating, typically towards the evening. This type of fasting can be leveraged for special occasions where you know there will be a lot of food. So that might be a snack at 4pm and a big(!) meal at 7pm, or two smaller meals.

Other variations

Obviously there are all the other permutations in between, e.g. 13:11, 14:10, 18:6, 19:5 etc, but the two most common TRE schedules are 16:8 and 20:4.

LONGER FASTS

Longer fasts are carried out such that you only eat a maximum of one meal during the day, and sometimes not even that . They can be carried out over a weekly, monthly, or yearly schedule, meaning they may be done once a week or twice a month, for example. You can also intersperse these longer fasts throughout your year if you plan to do daily fasts.

5:2 diet

In this diet, you 'fast' for 2 days of the week, only eating up to 500 calories on the 'fasting' days. You can eat normally on the other 5 days. I put the last fasting in quotes because on the 2 days where you are eating up to 500 calories, that isn't strictly fasting, but it still counts as you are likely to eat those 500 calories in one sitting. This is basically a diet because you're restricting and therefore counting calories two days a week.

24-hour fast

This type of fast is also confusingly known as the Warrior Diet. The key is to fast for 24 hours between each meal. If you eat dinner today at 7 pm, you will fast until 7 pm tomorrow night. Think of this as 23:1.

36-hour fast

The 36-hour fast is an extended version of the 24-hour fast, where you eat dinner on the first day, completely skip the next day, only drinking water or black tea/coffee that day, and eat breakfast on the third day.

Alternate day fasting

On this fast, you eat every other day. Just like the 5:2 variations, you have to keep your calories under 500 in one meal on the 'fasting' days.

Spontaneous fasting/ skipping meals

You simply skip meals if you are too busy or do not feel hungry.

WHY DIETS DON'T WORK

I've been talking about fasting vs dieting, so I think a section about diets is worthwhile, so that the two can be compared. Although dieting is popular, people sometimes move from diet to diet without finding something that works for them. You may have actually tried a diet or two and found out that they are not as effective as you would have liked, and that may be why you are reading this book right now. The most common problem that people face when dieting is that the weight that is frequently regained after the diet. A meta-study of 29 long term weight loss studies found that more than half of the weight lost during the dieting phase was regained within two years, and by five years more than 80% of lost weight was regained [1].

The biggest issue that many people face when they start diet plans is sustainability. Dieting is not easily sustainable over time, cannot easily be turned into a lifestyle choice, and relies on caloric restriction, which means you are hungry most of the time, so the body's negative feedback loops kick in so that you eat again.

About three years ago as an experiment I dieted for 9 months, eating around 1200 calories a day. It took a massive amount of willpower every day to stop eating what I wanted to eat, and it was hard not eating what the rest of the family was eating. My daughter was 16 at the time and I worried what sort of message it would send her. But I persevered and went from 160 pounds (73kg) to 130 pounds (59kg). Guess what weight I was 8 months later? Yep, 160 pounds.

Another big problem with diets is the calorie-counting part. Trying to track your calories is both very difficult and also inexact. If you've ever tried to use an app like MyFitnessPal for it, unless you individually weigh each piece of bread or knob of butter, then you are just guessing at the calories your buttered toast contained. And you can even end up eating the same thing again and again because selecting 'Yesterday's breakfast' for today's meal is way easier than scrolling through the app to try and find the size of your muffin you just ate..

So with dieting, you're hungry a lot of the time, you have to count calories, they are not sustainable for long periods of time and you don't get any of the health benefits associated with intermittent fasting that will be discussed later. Unlike with dieting, with intermittent fasting you don't have to count calories, you get lots of extra health benefits, and more importantly (for weight loss) after around 12 hours the body flicks a metabolic switch which doesn't happen during dieting as those reduced calories are still being consumed throughout the whole waking day. What happens when that switch is flicked is the next topic.

THE SCIENCE OF FASTING

A quick note before we start on this section. Whenever a scientific claim is made in this book, you will see a small number in brackets, e.g. [2], which will show you, at the back in the References section, which scientific journal the study came from. Please look these up, by using the shorter, simpler 'go' link listed after each reference, but which goes to the same place as the longer one. It just stops you from having to type the longer link into your browser.

To understand what's happening after you stop eating, it's helpful to break the process down into stages:

Fed State

While you are eating and until you have digested your meal completely, the food you have eaten gets broken down by enzymes in the body, starting with your saliva which breaks down carbohydrates, down into your stomach where both carbohydrates and protein are broken down, and then onto the small intestine where all three macronutrients (fat, protein and carbohydrates) are broken down by different processes and stored, or used for energy.

During this period, your blood sugar levels increase (from the breaking down of carbohydrates into simple sugars such as glucose), which in turn triggers more insulin to be secreted, as it is insulin that binds to the sugars so that it can enter your cells and be transformed into energy. Any extra that is not needed immediately is converted into glycogen and stored in your liver and muscles for use when the instant energy runs out. When the latter happens, the glycogen is converted back to sugar. The amount of time you are in the fed state often depends on the amount of carbohydrates you ingested in your last meal, but it is typically 3-4 hours.

A book on nutrition that is very good at explaining the basics is 'Understanding Nutrition', by Jason Houghton. It's not very long, but it breaks down the macronutrients into easily digestible chapters (geddit?) and explains the complicated processes in simple English.

Fasting State

In this state, your body sugar and insulin levels start to decline as they are used up in the form of energy, which in turn causes glycogen to be converted back to sugar. Once the latter falls below a certain level, the flicked metabolic switch we discussed earlier kicks in, namely the conversion of fat into energy (you may have heard the term 'ketosis'). This is done in multiple ways via complex processes such as lipolysis and gluconeogenesis. [2]

The point that fat starts to get converted into energy is around 12 hours. [3]

Now, just in case you missed it, I'll repeat that last bit.

The point that fat starts to get converted into energy is around 12 hours.

And that is why this chapter is called 'Why IF <u>will</u> work for you'. In a nutshell, when you fast for longer than 12 hours, your body will start converting fat and using it for energy, all without you asking. And the longer you can spend in the fasting state after 12 hours, the more fat you will burn. So provided you fast for more than 12 hours, you <u>will</u> lose weight.

This is one of the two reasons you'll succeed. The other will be discussed shortly.

Prolonged Fasting

18 hours after your last meal, you've completely switched to fat-burning mode and are generating significant ketones. Ketones promote cell and DNA repairs and are the fuel for our organs.

Within 24 hours, your cells are increasingly recycling old components and breaking down misfolded proteins linked to Alzheimer's and other diseases [4]. This is a process called autophagy. Autophagy is part of the cellular and tissue rejuvenation process that is responsible for removing damaged cellular components.

By 48 hours without calories or with very few calories, carbs, or protein, your growth hormone level is up to five times as high as when you started your fast [5]. Ketone bodies promote growth hormone secretion which helps decrease fat tissue accumulation, especially as people age.

By 72 hours, your body is breaking down old immune cells and generating new ones [6].

Through the different stages of fasting, you can see that the longer you fast the more your body benefits. To recap the above, you first start using fat as a fuel, but your body also starts removing old cells, increases your growth hormones and starts regenerating new cells. None of these benefits do you get with diets. And there are more.

BENEFITS OF FASTING

Although people come to intermittent fasting mainly as a weight-loss tool, there are many other health benefits to be gained from IF, some of which are discussed here:

1) It changes the function of some hormones, cells, and genes. During fasting human growth hormone increases (which has been shown to increase muscle mass and reduce body fat), and cellular repair augments through autophagy (discussed above), which is a protective house-keeping mechanism that eliminates damaged organelles (such as cell nuclei and mitochondria), misfolded proteins (from e.g. mutations), and invading pathogens (diseases etc). [7]

2) It can reduce insulin resistance, lowering your risk for type 2 diabetes. The more resistant to insulin your body is, the less sensitive it is to changes in sugar levels. As insulin is what allows sugars to enter cells to create energy, if there is not enough insulin to help convert the sugar, then the latter builds up in your bloodstream, which increases the risk of type 2 diabetes. [8]

3) It can reduce oxidative stress and inflammation in the body. Oxidative stress is one of the factors that contribute to aging and other chronic diseases. It occurs when there are too many free radical molecules in the body and not sufficient antioxidants to remove them. [9]

4) It can be beneficial for heart health, which may result in a longer lifespan. Fasting has been shown to improve different risk factors for heart disease, possibly due to weight loss which results in less stress being put on the heart. [10]

5) It may help in preventing cancer. This was found in animal studies and some human studies. In humans, it can also reduce the effects of chemotherapy. [11]

6) It may help prevent dementia. [12]

7-100) Asthma, Multiple Sclerosis, Arthritis etc etc. There are many, many more benefits, but it would be boring to list all of them, so we'll stop there. But if you want to read more on benefits, please consult the New England Journal of Medicine article accessed via this link (type it into your browser) tinyurl.com/nejmfast. After reading that, you'll wonder why you haven't been doing it for years already!

But don't just take my and the New England Journal of Medicine's word for it. Go to scholar.google.com (Google's index of scientific papers) and type 'intermittent fasting benefits' into the search bar to see how many scientific papers have been published on the topic.

Why do all these benefits come with IF ? A common belief is that until a couple of thousand years ago when humans stopped needing to be hunter-gatherers, daily life was a continual fast-feed cycle as food needed to be hunted and success rates varied day-to-day, depending on the season, amount of food sources, skill of hunters etc, and therefore our bodies are built to fast, and have health processes built in which are not being used any more now we can eat from morning till night. If that makes sense to you (as it does to me) then it's not surprising that all the health benefits and more will occur if you fast.

THE OTHER REASON INTERMITTENT FASTING WILL WORK FOR YOU

Let's say that in general you start eating when you wake up, then eat throughout the day, and go to bed an hour or three after you last ate (or drank) something. Most of us eat over a 12- to 14- hour window. So that would be three meals and a few snacks, along with soda, alcohol etc.

Now, imagine what happens when you compress those 12-14 hours down to say, 8. The reality is that you are unlikely to be able to fit in the time or stomach space to fill yourself with those same 3 meals, snacks and drinks in that reduced time-window. This would require you to eat a meal every 3.5 hours in order to finish the last one before the time-window ends. And to highlight the difference between possibly eating less on an IF regime and eating less on a caloric restriction/diet regime, on a diet you are hungry ALL THE TIME! Whereas on IF you may only be hungry for a couple of hours a day, and even then you might find that as a result of the health benefits you will incur, that actually you don't feel that hungry in your fasting window.

So it's this combination of possibly eating less and the fat-burning metabolic switch which will make you not only lose weight, but give you all the other health benefits listed above as well.

But to be clear, even if you continue to eat over say 8 hours what you used to in 14-16 hours, i.e. you take in the same calories you used to, the metabolic switch that kicks in over 12 hours will make you burn fat so you will still lose weight, only more slowly than if you ate less.

- I regularly fast but I eat 2500-3000 calories in my eating window as I am looking to put on muscle. For me, fasting keeps the fat off and gives me the benefits of autophagy, insulin sensitivity etc.

HOW MUCH WEIGHT CAN YOU LOSE?

Losing weight may not be an exact science but there are several scientific findings that show what works for some people. The same goes for intermittent fasting. According to the Harvard review carried out at their TH Chan School of Public Health [13]

"A systematic review of 40 studies found that intermittent fasting was effective for weight loss, with a typical loss of 7-11 pounds over 10 weeks."

More weight loss can be achieved by fasting for longer periods, but fasting for longer can be harder for some people (as we'll discuss in Chapter Three), so if you think of an approximation of a pound (or 0.5kg) per week then you won't be too far off. Now, as we'll also discuss later, the weight loss isn't always linear, and while the body is adapting to fasting in the first week or two you might not see any of those gains (or should I say losses!). But remember, what you will be gaining is all the other health benefits in that time, so it's time well spent.

Now you might be thinking that a pound a week isn't that much. But in 3 months (or 12 weeks), if you lose 12 pounds, and if you weighed 120 pounds at the start, that's 10% of your bodyweight! Of course you could lose more weight more quickly by drastically reducing the amount you eat, i.e. dieting, but there's three reasons you don't want to do that:

- It's not sustainable
- You'll just put it back on afterwards
- It's not healthy. Weight needs to come off slowly if you intend to keep it off

However, with IF once you get down to a weight that you are happy with, in the process you've mastered a tool that you can dip in and out of over the coming years should you decide to. IF should be seen as a lifestyle change rather than a temporary weight-loss measure, that will keep you healthy for the rest of your life.

WHO SHOULD NOT TRY INTERMITTENT FASTING?

Everyone wants to put their best foot forward and look and feel good, but it is not everyone that should try taking on IF. The following is a list of people who shouldn't, or should definitely consult their doctor before starting:

1) **You have a history of eating disorders.** Intermittent fasting is not recommended for anyone with an eating disorder because it can trigger a disordered pattern. It is crucial to listen to your body and to be mindful of what makes you feel healthy.

2) **You have digestion issues.** Undertaking IF can cause gastrointestinal distress if you already have digestion issues. Periods of fasting can cause constipation, indigestion, and bloating which spurs digestive issues.

3) **You have Type 1 diabetes.** IF may heighten the spikes and drops in blood sugar levels throughout the day. People with type 1 diabetes can go into a hyperglycemic state if they fast. If you are currently taking diabetes medicine you should consult your doctor before fasting and should be constantly monitored. The combination of diabetes medications and IF may cause dangerously low blood sugar levels.

5) **You're pregnant or breastfeeding.** If a woman is pregnant and they engage in IF, it may pose a threat to their fetus. When pregnant or breastfeeding the body requires an adequate calorie intake which will be interfered with by fast-

ing. If a woman is also trying to get pregnant IF is not advisable.

6) **You have a weak immune system or cancer.** If you were recently or are currently majorly ill, you should not engage in IF without consulting and clearing it with your doctor. Individuals with weakened immune systems or cancer require an adequate calorie intake.

You should consult your doctor before you start IF even if you do not fall under any of the above-mentioned categories. Finding out what is going on with you before and after the plan could capture the progress you are making.

Now, assuming that you don't fall into the above categories, let's talk about why you, as a woman over 50, should try IF.

2

---

3 REASONS WHY WOMEN OVER 50
NEED TO FAST

I wrote this chapter because other books allegedly for women over 50 didn't talk about how intermittent fasting could help their specific stage in life, and instead just quoted generic reasons why everyone should fast. So here are three reasons why women over 50 in particular should fast, and also importantly maybe <u>when</u> you shouldn't. These reasons are over and above the health benefits listed previously.

REDUCTION IN ESTROGEN LEVELS DECREASES YOUR METABOLIC RATE

According to research [14], changes in hormonal levels of estrogen cause various metabolic changes in the body, including less effective use of starches and blood sugar, which leads to an increase in fat storage, typically around the belly rather than hips and thighs. Storing more fat reduces your metabolic rate.

In addition, estrogen protects muscle mass, so when it is deficient muscle mass is lost, which in turn contributes to a slower metabolic rate [15].

So to counteract the increased storage of fat, an obvious way is to burn any increase through fasting.

INSULIN RESISTANCE MAY INCREASE

Before we get into this one, let's define what insulin is and what insulin resistance is.

Insulin is a hormone produced in the pancreas which regulates the amount of glucose in the blood. When glucose is circulating in the bloodstream, this causes insulin to be produced which binds to the cells' surfaces and allows the glucose to enter the cells to be turned into energy for use by those cells. Think of insulin as the key that opens the cell's door. Ideally the right amount of insulin is made, all the glucose is used by the cells and therefore glucose levels lower in the bloodstream, causing insulin levels to also decrease.

Insulin resistance occurs when the system is out of kilter. When a lot of sugar enters the bloodstream (e.g. after eating dessert) this causes the pancreas to produce insulin so the glucose can be ingested by your body's cells. Over time, your cells stop responding to the insulin, which has lots of negative effects such as the glucose not being used for energy as it can't enter the cell so it ends up being converted and stored as fat. In addition, the pancreas makes more insulin to try and make the cells respond and eventually the pancreas can't keep up. So even though the cells are crying out for glucose, the latter can't enter them and end up being stored as fat. Which results in you being tired and turning to carbohydrate-rich foods for fast energy, and so the cycle repeats.

So why do women over 50 need to care about this more than others? Again it comes back to levels of hormones that dictate insulin sensitivity. Hormones secreted by the thyroid and adrenal glands, as well as estrogen, all play a part in how sensitive your body is to insulin, so when these hormones fluctuate as they do in your 50s, the body will become more resistant to insulin's power of getting glucose into cells to create energy.

Again, for the same reason as mentioned above, whether extra fat is being laid down due to a slower metabolic rate or the body's inability to use the glucose it has consumed as a result of insulin resistance, fasting can more than offset any weight gains. [16]

EXERCISE

The two points above show why it's not surprising that women are likely to gain weight as they age, especially during perimenopause and menopause, even while eating and exercising the same amount as before. A slowing metabolic rate and a decrease in the body's ability to use up glucose efficiently ensures that fat will be laid down when once it wasn't.

So why can't we exercise to offset this weight gain? Surely we just need to walk a bit more every week and that should do it? In theory, yes, exercising can help you lose weight, and I heartily encourage you to exercise regularly, for various reasons. But here's the thing (or rather two things) :

1) one pound of fat contains ~3500 calories. So to burn off a pound of fat in theory you need to expend 3500 calories doing exercise. The body uses about 1300 calories a day just existing (breathing, thinking etc), so let's say you only need to burn off 2200 calories. Now, walking for an hour burns 200-300 calories, so taking the higher number you would need to walk about 7-8 hours a week to reach that goal, or an hour a day. A big commitment, especially if you have a job. And the more you eat, the more you'd have to walk.

2) finding the time to exercise is a challenge for most people, but women in their 50s have it especially hard. You might have a job, and if you do, given your seniority and experience the role will possibly be a demanding one. You may still have children at home who need your time as soon as you get home and before you go to work. And you may also have aging parents to look after as well. All these calls on your time are very stressful mentally, and given that you probably

put family first before thinking about yourself, the idea of going off for a couple of hours every day to exercise is not one you are likely to contemplate.

On the flip side, getting the body to do that work for you by fasting is much easier. And if you were to think about eating a bit less on a daily basis (which we'll talk more about in Chapter Four), then it's a lot easier to *not* eat 300 calories than to walk for an hour. If you can do both, then great.

WHEN YOU MAYBE SHOULDN'T FAST

One thing I would like to mention relates to those women who still have their period. In the last week before your period your hormone levels are at their lowest, and energy is needed to produce them. During this time you might be craving carbs, and that is no accident, it's your body's way of telling you that it needs the energy to produce estrogen and progesterone . So maybe either hold off on fasting for that week, or if you do feel good and are happy to keep going, then maybe make sure you're getting in the (good) calories.

OK, we've finally got to Step 1 of the program, namely learning about the different types of fasting protocols, and choosing one that's right for you to start with. Let's dive in!

This chapter covers the different types of IF and their pros and cons. Fasts can be broadly grouped into Time Restricted Eating (TRE), where you eat for X hours a day, and fast for the rest of the time, and longer fasts, i.e. 24 hours or more.

We'll discuss both below, and suggest which one to start with.

But before we do that let's discuss some factors that might influence your decision as to what types of IF and what windows will work for you.

3

STEP 1 - WHICH PLAN SHOULD I CHOOSE ?

This chapter covers the different types of IF and their pros and cons. Fasts can be broadly grouped into Time Restricted Eating (TRE), where you eat for X hours a day, and fast for the rest of the time, and longer fasts, i.e. 24 hours or more. We'll discuss both below, and suggest which one to start with.

But before we do that let's discuss some factors that might influence your decision as to what types of IF and what windows will work for you.

FACTORS AFFECTING YOUR DECISION

A Job

Having a job, and particularly one that requires entertaining clients or having work dinners may have an impact on which IF you pick. If you have breakfast meetings, or take clients out to dinner, that will steer you towards what time you will start or stop eating. If you work nights, then you'll have a different window from the rest of us. A job may also dictate what time you wake up and when you go to sleep, all of which goes into the 'when will I eat' equation. Picking a window that works for you and moving it around or pausing it is one of the many benefits of IF.

A Family

Eating meals together is an important part of family life, so if you gather round the table at 6pm every evening, again this will have a bearing on when you start eating during the day. Another factor related to eating with family members is that you may have teenage kids whose views on food are very impressionable, and you might want to avoid fasting when they're around in the evening. Again, what window(s) you pick can be tailored around your family so no-one else is affected by your choices.

Hungry When You Wake Up

Some people, like me, are often very hungry when they wake up. For me it's usually to do with when I ate the night before.

Oddly, the later I ate dinner the night before, the hungrier I am in the morning. I've found that finishing my evening meal earlier helps me not be so hungry the next morning, which is a bit counter-intuitive but that's just how I am. You might well be different.

Sleep

The longer you can sleep, the less fasting hours you have until your eating window starts, which can make fasting a breeze *if* you can sleep a long time. You may not have that luxury due to work, or you may not sleep so well, but it's worth mentioning just in case you do have the ability and capability to sleep long hours.

Ok, so let's get into the details of each type of fast.

TIME RESTRICTED EATING

16:8 Fasting

In the 16:8 intermittent fasting method, you only consume meals and calorific liquids during a window of 8 hours each day. For the following 16 hours (which includes sleep), you don't eat anything, but you are still allowed to drink water and other calorie-free beverages like black coffee or tea. Adding sugar or cream would start the eating cycle as they contain calories. Diet sodas are also not allowed as while calorie-free, they contain other ingredients that would stop the fasting cycle.

Depending on your preference, you can repeat this cycle as often as you'd like, from just once or twice a week to every day. You can also change which 8 hours you eat in along the way, so for example if you normally don't eat till midday but tomorrow you have a breakfast meeting then you just stop earlier on that day. If you have a breakfast meeting and a dinner meeting then you just skip that day. 16:8 fits into most lives and is typically seen as being less restrictive and more flexible than many other IF versions.

Let's say you're someone who feels they can't skip breakfast because you're hungry as soon as you wake up. In which case, pick a 7am-3pm window, or an 8am-4pm window.

If you're someone who likes to sleep in, maybe pick 12pm-8pm. If you eat as a family at 6pm, then pick 10:30am-6:30pm. If you work nights then maybe midnight-8am works for you.

Remember, you are not restricted to one window through-out, you can always change the window and even the length of the window depending on what's happening that day/week. So maybe do 10am-6pm one day and because you're going out to a restaurant the next day do 12pm-8pm then.

Many people choose to eat between the hours of 9 a.m. and 5 p.m. This gives them plenty of time to have a filling breakfast around 9 a.m., a typical meal around noon, and a light, early dinner or substantial snack around 4:30 p.m.

before beginning their fast. That may or may not work for you.

The ease and flexibility of 16:8 intermittent fasting is one of its key benefits as it can be tailored to fit your changing lifestyle, coupled with the fact that you get many health benefits in addition to weight loss. And the other good thing about 16:8 is that you can work up to it in small steps, which we'll discuss in Chapter Five. You may have by now guessed which type of IF I'm going to recommend at the end of this chapter!

So how many meals can you have a day on the 16:8 plan? The answer to this question depends on what you're trying to achieve. Some people doing a 12pm-8pm window skip breakfast, others start with breakfast at noon and end with dinner/supper and skip 'lunch', and others get three meals in that time. Obviously if you only eat twice then you're more likely to lose weight a bit more quickly, but some people (like me at the moment) are wanting to a) give their digestion system a bit of a rest and b) get the other health benefits (insulin sensitivity etc), so right now I'm eating three meals a day in my 8 hours. It depends on what your goal is, which we shall discuss more of in Chapter Five.

20:4 Fasting

This is the same as the above, apart from your eating window being half as long, i.e. 4 hours, and in this time you're probably only going to be able to eat one meal along with some snacks towards the end of the window. The benefits of this over 16:8 is that you are obviously in the fasting window for 4 more hours, which is 4 more hours of fat-burning, along with some autophagy kicking in. And you'll also be eating less, because it's difficult to eat 2000 calories in 4 hours (unless you eat nothing but cake and candy!).

But those extra benefits come at a cost. Going without food for 20 hours after you've been used to eating from 8am till 10pm is a real challenge, not forgetting living off half the calories you are used to. Also this might be more difficult to fit into your schedule, depending on your circumstances. So this is definitely one to work up to, or one that you can throw in once a week or once a month once you've been fasting for a while.

LONGER FASTS

One Meal A Day (OMAD)

OMAD constrains the eating window yet further down to around an hour, the time it takes to eat one (big) meal. It's basically 23:1 fasting, and comes with the same benefits and challenges as 20:4 fasting, so again, one for the future. A variation of this plan is the eat-stop-eat plan, where you do OMAD twice a week. So think of it as OMAD-lite.

5:2 Plan

Another IF plan includes 5:2, sometimes referred to as The Fast Diet. and popularized by Dr Michael Mosley, a British doctor and journalist.

The 5:2 plan is so-called because it allows for regular eating five days a week and restricts eating on the other two to 500–600 calories maximum each day. This plan is more of a lifestyle because there are no restrictions on what foods to consume or when to eat them. It is sometimes referred to as a diet in that on two of the days you are practicing caloric restriction, i.e. counting calories. The previous time-restricted eating plans do not require that.

Many people discover that this eating style is simpler to maintain than a conventional diet that restricts calories. Any two days of the week are acceptable as long as there is at least one day that is not a fasting day in between them. One typical weekly meal plan calls for eating regularly the other days of the week after a light meal on Mondays and Thursdays. Think of it as doing OMAD two days a week, but with the added complication of having to count the calories of that one meal.

On the two days when you only consume 500 calories, unless you spread those over a long period, you will definitely be getting some weight loss and other health benefits, and given you only have to watch what you eat twice a week, it's one of the easier plans to stick to. I have two friends that love 5:2, and do it a couple of times a year, like after the Christmas holidays for example, but they have been doing it for a while, so it's definitely one to consider, but again it maybe should be the third IF plan you try. We'll discuss easiest to hardest at the end of the chapter.

Alternate Day Fasting (ADF)

Another IF fasting strategy is alternate-day fasting (ADF). The fundamental concept is that you fast one day before eating everything you want the next day. By doing this, you are restricting what you eat 50% of the time.

You are permitted to have an unlimited amount of calorie-free beverages on days when you are fasting. As discussed already these would include water, unsweetened black tea and coffee. On a modified version of ADF, on fasting days, you're also permitted to consume roughly 500 calories, or 20–25% of your daily energy needs. That would basically be doing 5:2 but more like 4:3.

The modified form, with 500 calories on fasting days, was employed in the majority of investigations into alternate-day fasting. Although it is just as effective, this is thought to be considerably more maintainable than complete fasts on fasting days.

The ADF plan essentially means fasting for 32-36 hours at a time, as you stop eating in the evening on one day and don't start eating till the morning two days later. Fabulous for weight loss, autophagy and HGH levels, but it requires real mental commitment and the ability to live on around half the calories that you are used to. Again, one to try in the future once you've got comfortable with time-restricted eating.

SO WHICH IF PLAN SHOULD YOU START WITH FIRST?

As you've probably guessed, I think you should start with 16:8. Here's a list of 10 reasons why:

- You can work up to it
- You get both weight loss and other health benefits from doing 16:8
- It's easy to fit around your existing schedule
- You can still eat the same amount as before if you'd like
- No-one else in your life need be affected by you doing it
- You are much more likely to succeed doing this plan than longer ones
- It's one that you can stay on for all your life, if you choose.
- It can become your daily routine without you even thinking about it
- It's great training for longer plans, should you wish to try them

- It's very flexible, so you can change it around to suit your current circumstances

Longer plans can't claim all of the above. For beginners, they're harder to stick to due to the length of fasting windows, and every day is different so you have to remember where you are in the plan (e.g. which day of 5:2 are you on), or they may impact your family and social life.

Don't get me wrong, longer fasts are great to throw in every now and then to gain more of the fat-burning, autophagy and Human Growth Hormone benefits, but generally success is achieved by starting slow and working up to a task, not throwing yourself in at the deep end to see if you sink or swim. If you've fasted before or start with 16:8 and find it a breeze, then of course have a go at a longer fast if you want to.

If you want to work up to longer fasts, can I suggest that in order of ease, the path goes 16:8, then 20:4, then OMAD, then 36 hours, 72 hours etc.

So now is the time to complete step 1 in the program, namely to choose one of the plans listed above. If it's 16:8, then next you'll need to decide which 8-hour window you're going to start with. Is it 8am-4pm, 10am-6pm, 12pm-8pm, or another one? Remember this can always be moved to take into account personal circumstance. May I suggest that you take 5-10 minutes to have a really good think about which window works best for you and think through the next few days to see whether that window will work for them, or whether on one of the days the window will need to shift.

If it's a longer fast, then again play through the next few days to check that the fast fits in with what you'll be up to. If yes, then great, if not, the beauty of IF is that you can switch it up to suit your daily life, so choose another plan for the days when the longer fast isn't going to work.

So now we have talked about the different types of intermittent fasting and you've chosen one, let's move on to step 2. The next chapter is about whether you change your eating habits during the eating window.

4

STEP 2 — JUST IF OR IF+?

To start with, let's define what we mean by IF+. As we've discussed in earlier chapters, intermittent fasting is not a diet, and you can still lose weight by just eating what you ate previously, but all in a time window, so you eat the same as you always did, just in a time period of e.g. 8 hours. And if you've picked 16:8 as your plan, it's a great way to start your fasting journey. Success comes with small steps, and changing one thing at a time will make the likelihood of success much greater (Chapter Five is all about how to start).

There are also two other variables in addition to which fast/time window you've chosen, and they are a) how much you'll eat and b) what you'll eat. If you just decide to eat what you have always done but now in a time window, then that's regular IF. If however you decide to eat less or eat more healthily or both as well as time-restricted eating, then that's what I'm calling IF+.

Clearly the weight loss benefits will be greater if in addition to IF you also maybe eat less, or swap candy for veggies, but may I suggest you transition in stages, e.g. just IF (time-restricted eating) with what you currently eat, then maybe make some food substitutions, which will naturally reduce your calories as healthier food tends to have fewer calories than the not-so-healthy stuff, , and after that consider reducing your intake by maybe reducing portion sizes at each meal. But before we get into that in more detail, let's discuss the most important aspect of this journey.

YOUR WHY

The probability of achieving your goals will be greatly enhanced if you've worked out why you started on this journey in the first place, and what your goals are in terms of health. Being able to remind yourself every day why you are doing this will get you through any tough times you may encounter along the way.

So let's talk about goal setting. To start the process, you might first ask yourself 'why am I doing this?', and your answer might simply be 'to lose weight', or 'to feel healthier'. But that's not a sufficient motivator because it's not one that will spur you on on a daily basis. Instead, you then have to ask yourself 'why is that important to me?', and to each of your answers you need to keep asking yourself why that's important until you get to a tangible goal. For example:

Why do I want to intermittent fast? To lose weight
Why is that important to me? Because I don't like the way I look and feel
Why is that important to me? Because I want to feel younger again
Why is that important to mr? Because I want to live longer
Why is that important to me? Because I want to travel the world

Or

Why am I going to intermittent fast? To lose 20 pounds
Why is that important to me? Because I'm tired of being tired all the time
Why is that important to me? Because it stops me playing tennis
Why is that important to me? Because I love it and it not playing reminds me I'm getting older

In these two examples there are tangible goals, namely either being fit enough to travel the world or to play tennis. Envisioning yourself doing these things will help if/when the going gets tough.

Please take a few moments now to find your 'why', by doing the exercise above. Something that may help is the online tool 7levelsdeep.com which asks you what you want to do and then keeps asking you why it's important. It then saves your answers so you can keep a note of them. Maybe your end 'why' will be to play with grandkids, dance with your partner, learn to salsa or get back into your wedding dress. Whatever it is, knowing why you're doing this will help immensely. When you know your why, read on.

THE JOURNEY

Ok, now you know your 'why', you now have a goal that you can work towards, and you know exactly why you're on this journey. The next step is how you're going to get there, and how quickly (I'm hoping your goal is a medium- to long-term one, i.e. not 'get into this bathing suit for my vacation in 1 month', because as we've discussed before IF is a life-style, not a quick-fix. It's way more tortoise than hare).

Which means, we're going to be doing this over months and years, not days and weeks, and if you agree with me that making small changes to the plan each time is better than changing two or three things at once, then we have plenty of time to start with the easiest option, acclimatize to that, and then make one change, acclimatize to that etc. After all, like any scientific experiment, if you change two things at once, are the different results you get a result of changing the first thing, the second thing, or both? How will you know?

So my recommendation for the answer to the question 'IF or IF+?' is IF first, i.e. start with your existing meals compressed into a time window first, and then think about eating more healthily or skipping meals (IF+) after you've acclimatized to time-restricted eating. In the next chapter we'll discuss how you're going to start fasting, and the next steps once you get comfortable with the new regime.

5

STEP 3 — LET'S GO! (BUT DON'T MAKE THESE MISTAKES)

Ok, we're almost ready to go. I'm going to assume two things here, that a) we're going to work up to the 16:8 plan, and b) for now you're going to carry on eating what you do currently. Once you get comfortable with being on 16:8, we can start changing other parameters.

BIG MISTAKE #1

The first mistake is to not start slowly. I know this because I was one of those dummies who thought that eating one meal a day couldn't be so hard, so I started doing just that, eating one meal a day. The first day was great, and I didn't get that hungry. My dinner tasted fantastic, so I thought I'd just carry on. The next day was a bit tougher, but I got to dinner time and filled my face. It was on the morning of the third day that the crash hit me. I was so lethargic and found it difficult to get out of bed. I had a bit of brain fog, and a slight headache. But even I knew why I felt like crap. I had been eating considerably less calories than usual, and I wasn't giving my body any time to adjust from a 10:14 regimen to a 23:1! Of course that wasn't sustainable immediately. Please don't be a dummy like me.

BIG MISTAKE #2

The second mistake is to pick a start date when you've got lots of things on that week which will make it difficult or impossible for you to tighten your eating window by 2 hours. You need to start when you don't have lots of family or work commitments that could derail you before you even get going. Once you've started, when these commitments come along you can pause your fasting for those days or find a way to work around them, but that's a lot easier when you've been doing it for a while.

The third thing to mention is not a mistake, but a suggestion. Surrounding yourself with people who support your decision to try fasting and who don't try to knock you off course is very important. My partner was very skeptical when I first started, and each time the subject of fasting was brought up I was told it wouldn't work because I wouldn't stick at it or that I would just put the weight back on (they now admit that it worked and have started doing it themselves!). I think the reason for the reaction was that they felt it reflected badly on them because they weren't doing it. Who knows. Let's hope the people in your life are more encouraging

Anyway, I found my tribe online. I typed 'intermittent fasting' into Facebook, and joined 3 groups on the subject. I introduced myself in each and was overwhelmed by the positivity and warmth from complete strangers (they're not strangers any more). Whenever I needed some encouragement I would log on and read their inspirational stories, and I would recommend you do the same. It's a great way to stay on track, if some days your 'why' isn't enough.

Alternatively maybe you could find a friend to do this with? Lend them this book when you've finished reading it, and plan your journey together. They don't even have to be female or over 50 !

WORKING UP TO YOUR FIRST FAST

So first you have to work out on average how long your current eating window is. If you generally have breakfast at 7am and generally finish dinner at 8pm then your eating window is 13 hours, and in fasting ratios that would be 11(fasting):13(eating). If you start breakfast at 9am and finish dinner by 9pm that would give you 12:12. The plan is to make the left side number bigger than the right, i.e. you are trying to fast for longer than you eat, until you get to 16:8.

Now you know your ratio, add two hours to whatever the left number is and subtract 2 hours from the right, such that the total is still 24. So if your current ratio is 11:13, we are now aiming for 13:11, i.e. fast for 13 hours, eat for 11.

Once you've done that, either work back from when you are going to finish dinner or forward from when you plan to have breakfast. Whatever works for you and your work/family. So if you're now on a 13:11 schedule and you normally finish dinner by 7pm, that means not starting breakfast till 8am. If you have breakfast at 7am then you need to finish dinner by 6pm.

Stay on that plan for 3 days. This will give your body time to adjust. If you found it a breeze, step on up to the next 2-hour jump. So if you were on 13:11, move up to 15:9. If however you found it difficult then stay on the plan for now and remember the things you are about to read to help you get through the day. I hope what I'm about to say is an encouragement rather than a heart-sinker, but I found eating breakfast 2 hours later not that difficult. If I was occupied (more on this in a minute) then I often didn't even notice.

If you moved up to the next time restriction, stay on that one for 3 days, and then move up again until you hit 16:8. So you path may look something like this:

12:12 3 days
14:10 3 days
16:8 3 weeks

If those 3 day periods need to be extended so you and your body can get used to the new feelings and routine then that's not a problem. Remember, this is a marathon, not a sprint.

The reason I've put 3 weeks against 16:8 is that some people's bodies take a while to adjust to the new routine. A graph showing your weight loss over time will not be a straight line, especially at the beginning. Many things are happening in your body to adjust to the new routines (discussed in the Benefits section in Chapter One) and these adjustments don't happen overnight.

At this initial stage patience is a virtue. You may be one of the lucky ones who start losing weight very quickly, but my scales didn't budge for 2 weeks. I kept thinking 'maybe I need to increase the fasting window?' but my Facebook friends told me to be patient and they were right.

Hopefully you will find the transition process from 'before' to 16:8 relatively easy. But even if you do, the hacks below will make it even easier.

STAVING OFF HUNGER

There's no doubt about it, at some point in your fasting window you will get hungry. I get hungry when I don't sleep for long enough. When I wake up at 6:15 to help get my son off to school I often feel very hungry then, especially if I ate late the night before. I can't really be starving 7 hours later but my stomach thinks I am. The less sleep I get, the hungrier I feel. Which is where hack #1 comes in.

1. Sleep as long as you can - Whenever I'm fortunate enough to be able to sleep in, three things have changed compared to when I get 5-6 hours of sleep. The first is that I feel much better. The second is that I am no longer that hungry. And the third is that I've shaved another couple of hours off my fasting window. It's an obvious point, but the more you can sleep, the less time you spend awake while you're fasting, which means less time to feel hungry. Adding more time asleep might not be feasible for you (although we should all strive to sleep at least 7-8 hours), apart from maybe at weekends, but it's something to think about. Maybe start fasting when you go on vacation.

2. Drink lots of water/tea/coffee - there are three reasons for this. One is to fill your stomach up to reduce any hunger pains. The second is that we get a surprising amount of water from the food we eat, and if you get to the stage when you're cutting down on meals, then that lost water needs to be made up somehow if you don't want to be dehydrated. The third reason is that most of us don't drink enough water anyway. Just remember, it has to be plain water, or tea and coffee without any cream or sugar

or sweetener added. Anything added will take you
out of fasting.

3. Exercise - exercise does two things for fasting apart
from being good for you. It takes up time, and
anything that eats into the fasting window that stops
you thinking about food is a good thing, and it also
makes you less hungry anyway. My mind
concentrates on being tired after exercise, not on
being hungry.

4. Distract yourself - if you can, go to a movie, do a
jigsaw, or have a meeting in another building. When
I used to work in an office another lifetime ago, it
was always when I got bored that I started to get
hungry (usually around 10am!), but when work was
more involved or more fun I didn't think about food
so much.

5. Remember your 'why' - if all else fails, remember
that the best things in life don't come easy, and that
you have to work for them. If you can reframe those
hunger pangs as changes going on in your body that
are having a positive effect on your weight, your
mood and your longevity, then it's a price worth
paying. and hopefully you only have a couple of
hours to go till breakfast.

Hopefully, apart from the point about drinking more
water/tea/coffee, which you almost certainly will have to do,

you may find getting up to and staying at 16:8 a breeze. So please don't think you're going to be hungry all the time and fasting is going to be very difficult. For the majority of women it's not, especially after a few days when the body has got used to it. You might even see some benefits like weight loss and energy increase by then. But as I stressed before, this is way more tortoise than hare. Good things come to those who wait.

OTHER THINGS TO CONSIDER

Plan around your schedule

It's not difficult to plan around a busy schedule, but it does require a bit of thinking ahead. I use the diary in my phone to tell me when to start eating on the days that I can't start at midday and finish at 8pm. So for example if I'm going out to dinner tomorrow I assume I'll be eating till around 10pm, so I put a reminder in my phone to start eating at 2pm tomorrow. Some days there will be no solution, for example if you promised your kids that you would go out for breakfast, and that night you also have a party. In which case give yourself a break, have a day off, and get back on the horse tomorrow.

Don't compare yourself to others

Some people get easily discouraged when they compare themselves to other people. It is very easy to get caught up in comparing your journey and your plan to others, but you should avoid this. Your journey is unique to you. What works for you may not work for others and vice versa. Find a regimen that works best for you. Your body may respond differently when you fast at certain times or when you do a different fasting plan. This is because everyone has a different goal and metabolism.

RECAP

To recap the process:

1. work out your current eating window and subtract two hours from it
2. work out when you're going to start your fasting journey
3. keep to this new window for 3 days (or more if required)
4. subtract another two eating hours and stay on that regime for 3 days (or more)
5. move up to 16:8 and stay on it for 3 weeks minimum
6. remember the hacks to keep any hunger at bay

After you've been on 16:8 for three weeks you have a number of choices:

a. you could stick with this plan for the rest of your life, or until you hit a weight or health goal (benefits - weight loss,health)
b. you could keep this window but eat less in it, e.g.

skip breakfast (benefits - increased weight loss, health, saving money!)

c. you could eat less by restricting your time window to e.g. 18:6 or even 20:4 (benefits - even more weight loss and health benefits than b), saving money!)

d. eating more healthily in addition to the above options (benefits - all of the above but with even more health benefits)

We haven't really discussed option d) up to now despite the last chapter being all about healthy recipes and meal plans, and that was deliberate. When starting on any new path it can be easy to get overloaded with options and choices, and fall into analysis paralysis which results in no action being taken. So please, I would love you to try all the recipes at the back, but please get the mechanics of fasting down first before trying them out, unless you feel that you're finding the whole process easy (a lot of people do).

Ok, so now you are ready to start. Just follow the six steps shown above in the recap section and away you go. Do this for 4+ weeks, and then decide from the a) to d) points above what the next steps are going to be. You may decide that you're feeling good and you'd like to throw in a longer fast. You might decide to cut out one meal a day. You might decide to constrict your eating window even more. I did a 36-hour fast recently (essentially not eating for a whole day, and having breakfast at noon the following day) and my weight dropped by 3 pounds (about 1.5kg) in that time. A lot of that was due to not having a day's food in me, but longer fasting windows and/or less meals in the eating windows definitely speeds the weight loss process up. But it needs to be sustainable, so please make changes slowly to avoid crashing.

One last thing to mention is progress tracking. Obviously the easiest way to do this is by weighing yourself, but I know this can be a problem for some women. The issue is that other forms of tracking have a large margin of error, e.g. waist measurement, and any decreases will only show up over a longer time period. Seeing the number go down on the scale is a great motivator, and no one else needs to know what the number was that you started at. I weigh myself every day, and some days what I think the number is going to be and what it actually is are often quite different. I've learnt over time that a carb-rich diet the day before often increases my weight, but this is because carbs hold water well, so I often skip the weigh-in then as I know it won't be very reflective. I try to weigh myself at the same time every day, namely every morning just after I've got up and been to the bathroom. What I'm looking for is a trend, so providing the number at the end of the week is smaller than at the beginning, I'm happy. If it's not, then I keep going until it is. Basically, what I'm trying to say is, if you can face it, please weigh yourself before you start the journey, and then period-ically throughout.

The next chapters deal with exercise and fasting, myths about fasting and recipes/meal plans for when you've got 16:8 fasting nailed down.

YOUR CHANCE TO HELP OTHERS

In the first chapter of the book, we talked about why diets don't work, and it was one of the driving forces behind writing this book, because I wanted to convince people that there was an easier, more effective way to lose weight and keep it off.

If we're doing it right, we can learn from the mistakes of our past… and if we're really paying attention, we can learn from the mistakes of others too. I certainly have.

But mistakes aren't our only guiding force. We learn through studying, through watching, through practicing, through sharing our experiences… and this is where you as the reader have a chance to be part of the teaching process for the women of tomorrow. You can contribute in a small way by sharing the knowledge you have gained, either by word-of-mouth, or by lending this book to someone who may benefit. And for those women who you don't know who are also on the same path, you could help get this book on their radar.

By leaving a review of this book on Amazon, you'll show other women where they can find the guidance they're looking for.

Simply by telling other readers how this book helped you and what they can expect to find inside, you'll set them on the road to lasting health.

Thank you for your support.

Scan the QR code to leave a review!

6

BUT CAN I EXERCISE TOO?

This is a question I get asked a lot, and the simple answer is 'yes', but as with most questions relating to health, there are a number of nuances which we need to go over. The type of exercise, timing of your exercise, as well as what you're eating and how many calories you're eating all come into play.

To be clear, I would obviously advocate doing exercise in general, but if you're not doing any currently, and you feel that starting both fasting and exercising for the first time at the same time is a bit much, then I completely get it, and agree that taking on too much all at once might not be a great idea. Maybe start fasting first, and then move on to adding exercise once you're further along your fasting journey. In which case you can skip this chapter!

If you do currently exercise, depending on when you do it, you'll either be doing it in a fasted state or in a fed state. If you're planning to do 16:8 fasting starting around midday, then if exercising in the morning you will be in a fasted state, but anytime after midday you will be in a fed state.

Exercising on an empty stomach means your body is more likely to burn stored fat for energy instead of glucose from food. If I am planning to do a longer walk or get on the Peloton for 45 minutes I often do it in the mornings, 1) so I can get it over with (I get so bored on stationary bikes!) and 2) my body seems to be able to do longer, low-impact exercise on an empty stomach. Having said that, my numbers on the bike (power, speed etc) are not as good on an empty stomach as when I've eaten, as I don't have the ready source of energy available by exercising on an empty stomach.

I wouldn't, however, do a HIIT workout on an empty stomach, and would leave that until at least two hours after one of my meals. With those types of workouts the body generally needs more immediate energy than can be gained from burning fat, and you may find that your performance won't be up to the usual mark.

But as always, I may be different from you. And some days workouts go great and other days I can barely get through them. As always the secret is to listen to your body. Try exercising at different times of the day and see what works for you.

Just as a reminder of why you may want to exercise while fasting, here are some benefits.

BENEFITS OF WORKING OUT WHILE FASTING:

1. Increased fat loss: Fasted cardio may lead to increased fat loss, as the body burns stored fat for energy instead of glucose from food.
2. Improved insulin sensitivity: Exercise, especially when performed in a fasted state, may improve insulin sensitivity, which can help regulate blood sugar levels.
3. Enhanced metabolism: Working out in a fasted state can increase the body's metabolic rate and help it burn more calories throughout the day.
4. Better endurance: Training in a fasted state may improve endurance and performance during long-duration exercises.
5. Reduced inflammation: Exercise and fasting can both help reduce inflammation in the body, which is associated with a range of health issues.

It's important to note that the benefits of working out while fasted may vary between individuals and may depend on several factors, including the type and intensity of exercise, the duration of the fast, and overall health and wellness.

SOME THOUGHTS ON EXERCISE TYPES

If you are considering incorporating exercise into your fasting, I put down a few notes on strength training and yoga. I haven't done the same for cardio as I think you already know plenty about walking and running.

Strength Training

Strength training is a type of exercise that involves using resistance to build and maintain muscle mass. Some common forms of resistance used in strength training include weightlifting, resistance bands, and bodyweight exercises. The following are some key points about strength training, particularly for women over 50:

1. **Maintains muscle mass**: As we age, muscle mass naturally decreases, leading to a decline in strength and increased risk of falls and injuries. Strength training helps to counteract this loss of muscle mass, building and maintaining muscle mass, and improving overall strength.
2. **Supports bone health**: Strength training can also help support bone health and prevent the onset of osteoporosis, a condition in which bones become brittle and fragile. This is especially important for women over 50, who are at an increased risk.

3. **Improves balance**: Strength training can help improve balance, stability, and coordination, reducing the risk of falls and injuries.

4. **Boosts metabolism**: Strength training can increase the body's metabolic rate, helping to burn more calories and maintain a healthy weight.

5. **Increases energy**: Regular strength training can help boost energy levels, reduce fatigue, and improve overall mood.

It's also important to start slowly and gradually increase resistance and intensity over time to avoid injury and optimize results.

Exercise Routines

A few exercise routines could help you on this journey. These, done with constancy, would make you feel right as rain. I cannot overemphasize the role of exercises. Here are a few, but please don't try them without the requisite training and supervision, unless you're a gym pro:

1. Focus on compound exercises: Compound exercises, such as squats, deadlifts, and bench presses, target multiple muscle groups at once and can help maximize results.

2. Start with lighter weights: It's important to start with lighter weights and gradually increase resistance as you build strength and avoid injury.

3. Don't neglect form: Proper form is essential for maximizing results and avoiding injury, so it's important to focus on technique and use slow, controlled movements.

4. Focus on full-body workouts: To ensure all muscle groups are targeted, it's best to focus on full-body workouts that incorporate a variety of exercises.

5. Don't skip rest days: Rest days are essential for allowing muscles to recover and build strength, so it's important to allow for adequate recovery time between strength training sessions.

6. Incorporate cardio: Cardiovascular exercise, such as walking, cycling, or swimming, can help improve cardiovascular health and support overall fitness.

It's important to consult with a healthcare professional before starting a strength training program, especially if you have any pre-existing health conditions or injuries. A professional can help you determine the best approach for your individual needs and goals, including the type and frequency of exercises, resistance, and intensity.

Yoga

Yoga offers many health benefits for women over 50, including:

1. Improved Flexibility and Balance: Regular yoga practice can help improve flexibility and balance,

which can be especially important for women over 50 who may be experiencing age-related changes in these areas.

2. Reduced Stress and Anxiety: Yoga combines physical movements, deep breathing, and meditation, which can help reduce stress and anxiety levels. This is especially important for women over 50 who may be dealing with the physical and emotional challenges that come with aging.

3. Increased Strength and Endurance: Yoga involves a variety of postures that can help increase strength and endurance, especially in the core, arms, and legs. This can help women over 50 feel stronger and better able to tackle daily tasks.

4. Improved Sleep: Yoga has been shown to help improve sleep quality, which can be especially important for women over 50 who may be experiencing sleep difficulties.

5. Enhanced Mental Health: Regular yoga practice has been linked to improved mood, reduced symptoms of depression, and increased feelings of well-being.

Picking the right workout for your Intermittent Fasting (IF) plan depends on your goals and personal preferences. Here are three options to consider:

1. **Cardio**: Cardio workouts are great for boosting metabolism and burning fat. If you're looking to

maximize fat loss while practicing IF, this might be the best option for you.

2. **Strength Training**: Strength training helps build muscle and improve overall fitness. This is a great option for those who want to maintain or gain muscle while practicing IF. However, it's important to note that strength training may be less effective without adequate fueling, so it may be best to do it either before a meal or after breaking your fast.

3. **Yoga, Barre, and Low-Intensity Workouts**: Low-intensity workouts like yoga, barre, and Pilates can help improve flexibility, balance, and mind-body connection. They are a great option for those who want to avoid high-intensity workouts during their fasting periods or for those who are just starting out with IF.

Remember, everyone is different and what works for one person may not work for another. It's important to listen to your body and adjust your workout routine accordingly.

TIPS FOR WORKING OUT WHILE INTERMITTENT FASTING (IF)

1. Hydrate properly: Ensure to drink plenty of water before, during, and after exercising to avoid dehydration.

2. Listen to your body: If you feel weak or lightheaded during your workout, stop and eat a small snack.
3. Experiment to find what works best for you: Different approaches to IF may affect your energy levels differently, so it's important to find what works best for you.
4. Warm-up properly: Do a proper warm-up before starting your workout to prevent injury.

Specific Tips for maintaining balance and staying motivated

1. Start slow: Gradually increase the intensity and duration of your workouts to avoid injury.
2. Focus on balance: Incorporating balance exercises into your routine can help prevent falls and improve overall stability.
3. Strengthen bones: Weight-bearing exercises such as walking, weightlifting, and yoga can help strengthen bones and reduce the risk of osteoporosis.
4. Consider joint-friendly options: Low-impact exercises like swimming, cycling, and Pilates can be less stressful on joints.
5. Stay motivated: Find a workout buddy or join a class to stay motivated and on track with your fitness goals.

In summary, when exercising while practicing Intermittent Fasting (IF), it's important to properly hydrate, eat balanced meals before and after working out, listen to your body, and experiment to find what works best for you. It's also important to warm up properly to prevent injury. For women over 50, it's recommended to start slow, focus on balance, strengthen bones with weight-bearing exercises, consider low-impact options, and stay motivated through activities such as finding a workout buddy or joining a class.

Moving on to the next chapter, it's crucial to also consider other factors in addition to IF and exercise that contribute to a healthy lifestyle. I shall address some of these factors and debunk popular myths in the next chapter.

7

IF MYTHS

In this section I will tackle some of the most popular intermittent fasting myths. Let us begin by debunking one of the most well-known myths, namely that breakfast is the most important meal of the day.

1 – BREAKFAST IS THE MOST IMPORTANT MEAL OF THE DAY

You may have heard time and time again that breakfast is the most important meal of the day. Intermittent fasting (IF) can help your body learn to use fat and ketones as energy, allowing it to preserve muscle mass while metabolizing fat. Plus, the longer you fast, the less you will crave breakfast. IF is a great way to boost your health and get your body in its optimal state. In my experience what you eat and when you eat it are much more important than a label. I don't eat in the mornings and I feel great!

2 – THE BRAIN DOES NOT FUNCTION WELL WHILE FASTING

After several days, you come to understand the process of fasting. Everyone's starting point may differ but adapting to going without food for extended periods is universal. The brain can utilize glucose and ketones as energy sources, so it can continue to work optimally even when one of those sources has been used up.

3 – ALL INTERMITTENT FASTING IS THE SAME

There are several different types of IF plans as you have seen in the previous chapters. There is time restricted eating, one a meal a day fasting, and multiple day fasting. There are several variations that you can use to achieve your goal but remember to start out slow and to consult your nutritionist and doctor before diving headfirst into it.

4 – IF IS GOOD FOR EVERYONE

Intermittent fasting is quite a beneficial practice, but it may not be suitable for everyone. In Chapter One, we discussed who should and should not attempt IF. To recap, if you have a history with an eating disorder, an underweight physique, medical conditions that limit you or if you are either pregnant or breastfeeding - then intermittent fasting is not recommended for you.

5 – INTERMITTENT FASTING MAKES YOU OVERINDULGE

Contrary to popular belief, eating after fasting does not necessarily lead to overeating. If you're fasting then you know that eating too much will work against your goals. What IF does do is make you appreciate your food more. The longer the fast, the more you savor those first mouthfuls.

6 – FASTING IS HARMFUL FOR OUR BRAINS

The faster your body adjusts to fasting the more resilient your cells become. Our brains and bodies can last for many days without eating if we put our mind to it. Over time ketones become the predominant source of energy when you fast which makes it possible for you to experience mental clarity while fasting. Ketones have allowed humans to live through times of famine and limited food availability.

7 – FASTING CAUSES CHANGES IN MOOD

At the beginning of a fast, some people may experience fluctuations in mood, but once their body adjusts to the regimen, those changes will even out, and their emotions will become regulated. If you have a positive attitude and are determined, your body can fast for extended periods.

8 – IF IS NOT SUSTAINABLE

Most individuals think of intermittent fasting as a type of diet, and thus consider it to be unsustainable. However, this is simply not the case. With IF, you can easily manage your food intake without having to continuously fight cravings. Once you get accustomed to your routine, you will no longer be preoccupied with food during your fasting window. IF is completely flexible and thus sustainable.

Ok, on to recipes. To be clear, these are only provided in case you're looking to eat a bit more healthily, and ideally once you have been fasting a bit already and are comfortable with the changes you may have observed while doing so.

8

RECIPES AND MEAL PLANS

This chapter contains over 50 recipes, broken down into snacks, breakfast lunch and dinner, along with two suggested meal plans. One way to view them all is in the table of contents of this book. Hope you find some that you like.

SNACKS

All of the following recipe measurements are according to US units.

Spicy Chocolate Keto Fat Bombs

INGREDIENTS
2/3 cup coconut oil

2⁄3 cup smooth peanut butter

1⁄2 cup dark cocoa

4 (6 g) packets stevia (or to taste)

1 tablespoon ground cinnamon

1⁄4 teaspoon kosher salt

1⁄2 cup toasted coconut flakes

1⁄4 teaspoon cayenne (to taste)

DIRECTIONS

1. In a double boiler pour the peanut butter, coconut oil, and cocoa powder and set the boiler on top of a pot of simmering water. As the ingredients melt, whisk everything together until everything has melted and the mixture is smooth.
2. To the mixture add the salt, cinnamon, and stevia for taste and mix into the mixture.
3. You can distribute the mixture into a silicone mini muffin tray. Another option is to use liners and distribute the mixture among them in a mini muffin tin.
4. Sprinkle some coconut and cayenne on top, then put the tray in the freezer until the mixture is firm. This usually takes around 30 minutes.

Cauliflower Popcorn

INGREDIENTS

1 head cauliflower

4 tablespoons olive oil

1 teaspoon salt, to taste

DIRECTIONS

1. To start, preheat your oven to 425 degrees.
2. Prepare the cauliflower by removing the core and thick stems from the head, and then cutting the florets into ping-pong ball-sized pieces.
3. In a large bowl, whisk together some olive oil and salt, and then toss in the cauliflower pieces until they're evenly coated.
4. For easy cleanup, you can line a baking sheet with parchment paper before spreading the cauliflower pieces on it. Roast the cauliflower for about an hour, turning the pieces 3 or 4 times, until they're mostly golden brown. (Note: The more caramelization occurs, the sweeter the cauliflower will taste).
5. Once the cauliflower is done, serve it immediately and enjoy!

Vegan Coconut Kefir Banana Muffins

INGREDIENTS

2 cups all-purpose flour

1 cup granulated sugar

1 cup unsweetened dried shredded coconut

2 teaspoons baking soda

1 teaspoon baking powder

1/2 teaspoon salt

2 ripe bananas, mashed

1 1/2 cups pc dairy-free kefir probiotic fermented coconut milk

1/4 cup cold-pressed liquid coconut oil

1 teaspoon vanilla extract

DIRECTIONS

1. Preheat your oven to 350°F (180°C) and lightly coat a 12-count muffin tin with cooking spray.
2. In one bowl, whisk together the flour, sugar, coconut, baking soda, baking powder and salt. Set aside.
3. In a larger bowl, whisk together the bananas, kefir, coconut oil and vanilla extract until everything is incorporated. Pour the wet ingredients into the dry ingredients and fold in until no streaks of flour remain.

4. Evenly divide the batter among the prepared muffin tin and bake for about 30 minutes or until a toothpick inserted into the center of a muffin comes out clean. Let cool for 15 minutes before transferring to a cooling rack.

Chef's tip: To freeze these muffins, let them cool completely on a rack, then individually wrap each muffin in plastic wrap or foil before transferring them to an airtight container or resealable freezer bag and freezing for up to one month. Thaw in the fridge overnight or microwave straight from frozen for about 20 to 30 seconds.

Trail Mix

INGREDIENTS
cup almonds (raw)
1 cup sunflower seeds (raw)
1 cup raisins
1/2 cup dried apricot (unsulphured, chopped)
1/4 cup flaked coconut (optional)
1/4 cup chocolate (optional) or 1/4 cup carob chips (optional)

DIRECTIONS

Mix everything together in a container with a lid and shake it well until everything is thoroughly mixed. Store in an airtight container and place in the fridge or freezer to retain essential fatty acid properties.

Caramelized Onion-Cranberry Cream Cheese Bites

INGREDIENTS

1 tablespoon butter

2 cups thinly sliced sweet onions

1/4 cup balsamic vinegar

1/2 cup cranberries, coarsely chopped

1 tablespoon sugar

1/2 teaspoon salt

1/2 teaspoon grated orange rind

16 whole wheat crackers

8 ounces low-fat cream cheese

DIRECTIONS

1. Melt butter in a large pan over a medium heat, then add onions when butter melted, and sauté for around 15 minutes or until golden. Stir in vinegar and the rest of the ingredients, and stir occasionally, for 2-3 minutes or until liquid is reduced to about 2 tablespoons.

2. Spread 16 whole grain crackers each with 1 1/2 teaspoons cream cheese, and top each with 1 tablespoon of the sauce. Garnish with parsley.

Pizza Meatloaf Cups

INGREDIENTS

1 egg, beaten

1/2 cup pizza sauce

1/4 cup seasoned bread crumbs

1/2 teaspoon italian seasoning

1 1/2 lbs ground beef

1 1/2 cups shredded part-skim mozzarella cheese

DIRECTIONS

1. In a bowl, combine the egg, bread crumbs, Italian seasoning and pizza sauce and mix into a paste.
2. Fold beef into the mixture and mix well.
3. Divide the beef mixture equally into 12 greased muffin cups.
4. Press the mixture into the bottom and up the sides.
5. Fill the center with cheese.
6. Bake at 375°F/190°C for 15 minutes or until the meat is no longer pink.
7. Serve immediately with additional pizza sauce and cheese if desired.
8. Or cool, place in freezer bags and freeze for up to 3 months.

Cheese Bites

INGREDIENTS

2 lbs sharp cheddar cheese, shredded

2 cups unsalted butter, softened

5 cups all-purpose flour

1 teaspoon salt

1/2 teaspoon cayenne pepper

DIRECTIONS

1. Combine the cheese, flour, butter, cayenne pepper and salt in a large bowl, and knead into a dough.
2. Roll the dough into 1 inch balls and place on an ungreased baking sheet.
3. Preheat the oven to 425°F/220°C.
4. Bake for 13-15 minutes.

Smoked Salmon Spread

INGREDIENTS

12 ounces cream cheese, at room temperature

1/3 cup sour cream

1 tablespoon fresh lemon juice

6 dashes Tabasco sauce

3 scallions/spring onions, white and green parts, thinly sliced

3 tablespoons capers, rinsed and drained

8 ounces smoked salmon, coarsely chopped

3 tablespoons chopped fresh dill or 1 tablespoon dried dill

fresh ground black pepper

fresh dill, for garnish

crackers or breadstick, for serving

DIRECTIONS

1. Puree the cream cheese, lemon juice, sour cream and tabasco in a mixer.
2. Add the scallions/spring onions, salmon, capers, chopped dill and pepper, and pulse to blend.
3. Garnish with the dill and serve chilled or at room temperature with crackers.

Bacon-Wrapped Scallops

INGREDIENTS

6 slices of bacon

12 sea scallops (if very large, cut in half)

3 tablespoons butter

1 tablespoon minced garlic

1/3 cup chicken broth/stock

DIRECTIONS

1. Cut each bacon strip in half, width-ways.
2. Wrap a piece of bacon around each scallop and secure with a toothpick.
3. Place the wrapped scallops on a baking sheet.
4. Broil/grill 6 inches from heat for 3 minutes each side, or until bacon is crisp.
5. In a small pan, melt the butter, then add the garlic and saute for 1 minute.
6. Add the chicken broth/stock and bring to a boil.
7. Cook for 2 minutes.
8. Place scallops in a large bowl and pour the broth over, tossing gently to coat.
9. Serve immediately.

Toasted Ravioli

INGREDIENTS

2 dozen cheese ravioli or 2 dozen other filled ravioli, thawed if frozen

2 eggs, lightly beaten

1 cup Italian seasoned breadcrumbs

parmesan cheese

vegetable oil (for frying)

marinara sauce (for dipping)

DIRECTIONS

1. Cook the ravioli in boiling salted water until they float to the top, and then drain.
2. Set aside to cool.
3. Heat vegetable oil in a pan so that the oil is at least 2" deep, to 375°F/190°C.
4. Dip the ravioli in the beaten egg, and then coat in the breadcrumbs.
5. Fry in batches until golden brown, roughly 5 minutes, and then drain.
6. Sprinkle the hot ravioli with parmesan cheese.
7. Heat marinara sauce and set aside in a serving bowl.
8. Serve ravioli with dipping sauce.

Zucchini Bites

INGREDIENTS
1 tablespoon olive oil
1 onion, finely chopped
3 slices rindless bacon, finely sliced
1 large carrot, grated
1 large zucchini, grated
3 eggs
1 cup cheese, grated
1/4 cup cream
1/2 cup self rising flour

DIRECTIONS

1. Heat the oil in a large pan and saute the onion for 8 minutes over a medium heat, stirring occasionally.
2. Add the bacon and fry until it starts to brown.
3. Add the carrot and zucchini and cook for about 2 minutes.
4. Transfer the mixture to a bowl to cool.
5. Beat the eggs, cream and cheese together, and season to taste.
6. Stir the egg mixture into the cooled zucchini mixture. Stir in the flour.
7. Grease and flour little muffin/bun tins. Spoon mixture into the holes.
8. Bake at 180°C/350°F/Gas 4 for 15-20 minutes.

Hot and Spicy Peanuts

INGREDIENTS

2 teaspoons vegetable oil

2 cups unsalted peanuts

2 teaspoons chili powder

1/4 teaspoon ground red pepper (cayenne)

1/2 teaspoon garlic salt

DIRECTIONS

1. In a pan, heat the oil over a medium heat. Stir in the peanuts, chili powder, and red pepper.
2. Cook and stir for 2 minutes or until the peanuts are warm. Drain well on paper towels.
3. Sprinkle the garlic salt over the peanuts and toss to combine. Cool completely.
4. May be stored in a tightly covered container at room temperature.

BREAKFAST

Summer Berry Crisp

INGREDIENTS
FRUIT
1 (16 ounce) bag cherries or (16 ounce) bag blueberries
1 (7/8 ounce) box jello sugar-free vanilla pudding mix, cook and serve
1 teaspoon cinnamon
1/2 teaspoon nutmeg
1/4 cup nonfat milk

CRISP
1 1/2 cups old fashioned oats
1/2 cup Splenda sugar substitute
8 ounces plain fat-free yogurt

1 teaspoon almond extract

DIRECTIONS

1. Lightly coat an 8X8 baking dish with cooking spray.
2. Place the fruit ingredients in the pan and stir together.
3. Mix up the crisp topping ingredients in a separate bowl.
4. Sprinkle this mixture over the top of the berry mixture.
5. Bake at 350°F for forty to forty-five minutes or until the topping becomes crunchy.

Peach Berry Smoothie

INGREDIENTS

1 cup frozen peaches
1/4 cup coconut milk (adjust for thicker or thinner smoothie)
1/2 cup Greek yogurt
1/2 teaspoon almond flavoring

DIRECTIONS

1. In a blender on high speed, blend together peaches and almond flavoring.

2. Check the consistency and modify to your desired texture. Add more milk for a thinner texture and more peaches for a thicker texture.
3. Garnish with chia seeds, berries, and slivered almonds for an aesthetically pleasing topping. Enjoy!

French Vanilla Almond Granola

INGREDIENTS

3 1/2 cups old fashioned oats (not quick)

1/2 cup sliced almonds

1/2 cup water

1/2 cup natural cane sugar

1/4 teaspoon salt

1/4 cup organic canola oil or 1/4 cup grapeseed oil

1 tablespoon vanilla extract

DIRECTIONS

1. Preheat the oven to 200 degrees Fahrenheit. Then, take a large, rimmed baking pan and line it with parchment paper.
2. In a large bowl, combine the oats and almonds.
3. In a small saucepan over medium heat, add the sugar, salt, and water. Stir until the sugar has dissolved. Take the pan off of the heat and mix in the canola oil and vanilla extract. Pour this mixture into the bowl

containing oats and almonds and stir everything together.

4. Pour the mixture out onto the pre-lined baking pan, and bake for two hours or until it's dry to the touch. Don't stir it! Once finished cooking, let it cool before breaking it apart into chunks. Finally, store in an airtight container.

Poached Eggs and Avocado Toast

INGREDIENTS

4 eggs

2 ripe avocados

2 teaspoons lemon juice (or juice of 1 lime)

4 slices thick bread

1 cup cheese (grated, edam, gruyere or whatever you have on hand)

salt & freshly ground black pepper

4 teaspoons butter (for spreading on toast)

DIRECTIONS

1. Poach some eggs with your preferred method.
2. Cut the avocados in half and get rid of the pits.
3. Use a spoon to scoop out the fruit from the skin and put it in a bowl with the lemon or lime juice, salt, and pepper.

4. Mash the mixture with a fork until it's relatively smooth.

5. Toast some slices of bread and spread butter on each one.

6. Smear the avocado mix onto each of the buttered toasts, then put a poached egg on top of each one.

7. Sprinkle some grated cheese as a finishing touch, then serve as soon as possible. You can also have fresh or grilled tomatoes as an accompaniment.

The Easiest Hard-boiled Eggs

INGREDIENTS
6 large eggs

DIRECTIONS

1. Put your eggs into a medium sized pot and pour water until it is an inch above the eggs. Put the pot on a stove that is on high heat.

2. Once it is boiling, remove the pot from the stove and place the lid on the pot, Let the covered pot sit for 18-20 minutes.

3. Pour cold water into the pot with the hot water, to flush out the hot water. To get the water out faster, hold the pot slightly slanted. Once the water in the pot is cold, let the eggs sit in the cold water for a minute or two. They are now easy to peel.

NB: You can peel the eggs under running water over a colander, so catch the egg peels. If you are putting the eggs in a salad you can place the peeled eggs on a paper towel to remove excess moisture. To keep the eggs fresh for 4-5 days, you can place them into a bowl with cold water, cover it and refrigerate.

Avocado Quesadillas

INGREDIENTS
2 vine-ripe tomatoes, seeded and chopped into 1/4 inch pieces
1 ripe avocado, peeled, pitted, and chopped into 1/4 inch pieces
1 tablespoon chopped red onion
2 teaspoons fresh lemon juice
1/4 teaspoon Tabasco sauce
salt and pepper
1/4 cup sour cream
3 tablespoons chopped fresh coriander
24 inches flour tortillas
1/2 teaspoon vegetable oil
1 1/3 cups shredded monterey jack cheese

DIRECTIONS

1. Combine the tomatoes, avocado, onion, lemon juice and Tabasco sauce in a small bowl, seasoning with salt and pepper to taste.
2. In a separate bowl, mix together the sour cream with coriander, salt and pepper.
3. Put tortillas on a baking sheet and brush the tops with oil.
4. Place the tortillas 2 to 4 inches away from the heat source and broil until slightly golden.
5. Sprinkle some cheese over the tortillas and place them back in the broiler until the cheese melts.
6. Divide the avocado mixture between two tortillas, topping each with one of the remaining tortillas so that the cheesy side is down, creating two quesadillas.
7. Slice each quesadilla into four wedges and top each wedge with a spoonful of sour cream mixture before serving warm.

Egg and Veggie Scramble

INGREDIENTS
1/2 tablespoon (30 mL) coconut oil
roughly 1 cup (70–150 grams) fresh or frozen vegetables of your choice (I like sliced mushrooms)
2 eggs, beaten

salt and pepper

DIRECTIONS

1. Place a skillet on the stovetop and switch the heat to medium.
2. Throw in your preferred vegetables and let them simmer until they get a nice golden-brown color. If you're using frozen veggies, these will need a few extra minutes.
3. Then, add in your eggs, season with a pinch of salt and pepper, and keep stirring all the while so they don't burn.
4. Once the eggs have cooked through, take the pan off the heat and serve your egg dish hot.

Bacon and Eggs

INGREDIENTS
2 slices bacon
2 eggs
salt and pepper

DIRECTIONS

1. Begin by cooking the bacon in a frying pan over medium heat until it reaches the desired crispness.

2. Move the bacon to a plate, then add the eggs and season with salt and pepper.

3. Leave the yolks intact if you like your eggs runny and don't forget to flip them when the whites on the bottom have set. If you want fully cooked yolks, break them in the pan. Once the entire white has set, remove eggs from heat.

Overnight Chia Pudding

INGREDIENTS
2 tablespoons (24 grams) chia seeds
3/4 cup (180 mL) unsweetened milk of your choice
liquid stevia drops (or your preferred sweetener)
berries for topping (strawberries and raspberries are low in carbs)

DIRECTIONS

1. In a mason jar with a lid, pour all your ingredients except the berries inside and close it up with the lid. Refrigerate the mixture overnight.

2. The next morning you can add the berries and enjoy your meal.

LUNCH

Bunless Butter Burger

INGREDIENTS
1/2 tablespoon (7 grams) butter
1 preformed hamburger patty
salt, pepper, and Worcestershire sauce

DIRECTIONS

1. Melt butter in a skillet over medium-high heat.
2. Place the hamburger patty in the skillet and season it with salt, pepper, and Worcestershire sauce.
3. After a few minutes, turn the patty over and season the other side. Cook it through until there is no pink in the middle or until the juices run clear.
4. Adorn the burger with your favorite low carb toppings and serve with a side salad to make it a full meal.

Grilled Lemon Salmon

INGREDIENTS
2 teaspoons fresh dill
1/2 teaspoon pepper
1/2 teaspoon salt
1/2 teaspoon garlic powder

1 1/2 lbs salmon filets

1/4 cup packed brown sugar

1 chicken bouillon cube, mixed with

3 tablespoons water

3 tablespoons oil

3 tablespoons soy sauce

4 tablespoons finely chopped green onions

1 lemon, thinly sliced

2 slices onions, separated into rings

DIRECTIONS

1. Generously season the salmon with dill, pepper, salt and garlic powder.
2. Put the salmon in a shallow glass dish.
3. Mix together sugar, chicken bouillon, oil, soy sauce and green onions.
4. Saturate the fish with this marinade.
5. Refrigerate for an hour, turning it once.
6. Discard the marinade and place the salmon on a preheated medium heat grill.
7. Lay some slices of lemon and onion on top of the fish and cover the grill.
8. Cook for fifteen minutes or until cooked through.

Avocado Waldorf Chicken Salad

INGREDIENTS

about 1 cup (140 grams) shredded cooked chicken (you can use a rotisserie chicken for convenience)

1 green apple, cored and diced

5 seedless grapes, quartered

2 celery stalks, finely chopped

1 ounce (28 grams) crushed walnuts

1 large avocado, pitted, peeled, and smashed

1 teaspoon (5 mL) lemon juice

salt and pepper

DIRECTIONS

1. In a medium bowl, mix together chicken, apple, grapes, celery, and walnuts.
2. Fold in the avocado and squeeze lemon juice over the top. Blend until the avocado has enveloped all the ingredients.
3. Sprinkle in salt and pepper to taste.

Veggie-Packed Cheesy Chicken Salad

INGREDIENTS

1 cup cooked boneless skinless chicken breast, cubed

1/4 cup celery, finely chopped

1/4 cup carrot, shaved into ribbons

1/2 cup Baby Spinach, roughly chopped

2 1/2 tablespoons fat-free mayonnaise

2 tablespoons nonfat sour cream

1/8 teaspoon dried parsley

2 teaspoons Dijon mustard

1/4 cup reduced-fat sharp cheddar cheese, shredded

DIRECTIONS

1. Combine the ingredients in a bowl and cover them completely with the mayonnaise.
2. Place the bowl in the refrigerator and let it cool for half an hour, or even better, prepare it the night before. Serve and enjoy!

Cobb Salad with Brown Derby Dressing

INGREDIENTS

1/2 head iceberg lettuce

1/2 bunch watercress

1 bunch chicory lettuce

1/2 head romaine lettuce

2 medium tomatoes, skinned and seeded

1/2 lb smoked turkey breast

6 slices crisp bacon

1 avocado, sliced in half,seeded and peeled

3 hard boiled egg

2 tablespoons chives, chopped fine

1/2 cup blue cheese, crumbled

DRESSING

2 tablespoons water

1/8 teaspoon sugar

3/4 teaspoon kosher salt

1/2 teaspoon Worcestershire sauce

2 tablespoons balsamic vinegar (or red wine vinegar)

1 tablespoon fresh lemon juice

1/2 teaspoon fresh ground black pepper

1/8 teaspoon Dijon mustard

2 tablespoons olive oil

2 cloves garlic, minced very fine

DIRECTIONS

1. Garnish with chives, and arrange on the table.
2. Toss the salad with the dressing just before serving, and use chilled salad bowls. Serve with fresh French bread.
3. To make the dressing, blend all ingredients except the olive oil in a blender.
4. Add the oil gradually while running the machine, until blended well. Refrigerate the dressing until ready to use.

*REMEMBER: The salad should be as cold as possible when served.

Vegan Fried 'Fish' Tacos

INGREDIENTS

14 ounces silken tofu

2 cups panko breadcrumbs

1/2 cup plain flour

1/2 teaspoon salt

1 teaspoon smoked paprika

1/2 teaspoon cayenne pepper

1 teaspoon ground cumin

1/2 cup non-dairy milk

vegetable oil, for frying

1/4 head cabbage, finely shredded

1 ripe avocado

8 small tortillas

vegan mayonnaise, to serve

PICKLED ONION

1 red onion, peeled, finely sliced

1/4 cup apple cider vinegar

1 tablespoon sugar

1 teaspoon salt

DIRECTIONS

1. Gently press the tofu with a few sheets of kitchen
   roll to remove extra moisture. Using a knife, cut the
   tofu into roughly 1-inch chunks. They don't need to

be perfect; it's more visually appealing if it looks slightly imperfect.

2. In one wide shallow bowl, fill it with breadcrumbs.

3. In another wide shallow bowl, fill it with flour, salt, smoked paprika, cayenne and cumin.

4. Mix them together and then pour the milk in a third wide shallow bowl.

5. Take the tofu and coat each chunk first in the flour, then in the milk, then finally in the breadcrumbs. Place them on a baking sheet.

6. Fill a deep frying pan with about 1/2 inch of vegetable oil. Warm it up over a medium heat until it starts to bubble and brown when a breadcrumb is dropped in. Carefully add the chunks of breaded tofu to the oil and fry until golden underneath; flip them over and cook until golden all around. Transfer to a baking sheet lined with kitchen roll to drain any excess oil. Repeat this process with the rest of the tofu.

FOR THE PICKLED ONION:

1. Bring the apple cider vinegar, salt and sugar to a boil in a small saucepan. Put the thinly sliced red onion in a bowl or container and pour the hot vinegar mixture over it. Let it sit for at least half an hour so that it can steep and become pink.

2. Serve warm fried tofu in tortillas (which you can preheat your tortillas on the gas rings of your stove- if you have one), pickled onion, vegan mayo, avocado slices and shredded cabbage.

Mediterranean Chicken Breasts with Avocado Tapenade

INGREDIENTS
4 boneless skinless chicken breast halves
1 tablespoon grated lemon peel
5 tablespoons fresh lemon juice, divided
2 tablespoons olive oil, divided
1 teaspoon olive oil, divided
1 garlic clove, finely chopped
1/2 teaspoon salt
1/4 teaspoon ground black pepper
2 garlic cloves, roasted and mashed
1/2 teaspoon sea salt
1/4 teaspoon fresh ground pepper
1 medium tomatoes, seeded and finely chopped
1/4 cup small green pimento stuffed olive, thinly sliced
3 tablespoons capers, rinsed
2 tablespoons fresh basil leaves, finely sliced
1 large Hass avocado, ripe, finely chopped

DIRECTIONS

1. Gather the ingredients for the marinade: 2 tablespoons of lemon peel, 2 tablespoons of lemon juice, 2 tablespoons of olive oil, garlic, salt and pepper. Place the chicken with the marinade into a sealable plastic bag, seal it, and refrigerate for 30 minutes.

2. In a bowl, combine the remaining 3 tablespoons of lemon juice, roasted garlic, 1/2 teaspoon of olive oil, sea salt and freshly ground pepper. Once combined, mix in the tomato, green olives, capers, basil and avocado. Set aside.

3. Take the marinated chicken out of the bag and discard the leftover marinade. Cook it over medium-hot coals for 4 to 5 minutes per side or until it is done to your liking.

4. Serve with Avocado Tapenade.

Shredded Brussels Sprouts with Bacon & Onions

INGREDIENTS

2 slices bacon

1 small yellow onion, thinly sliced

1/4 teaspoon salt (or to taste)

3/4 cup water

1 teaspoon Dijon mustard

1 lb Brussels sprout, trimmed, halved and very thinly sliced

1 tablespoon cider vinegar

DIRECTIONS

1. In a large skillet on medium heat, cook the bacon until it's crisp (5-7 minutes). Drain the bacon on paper towels and crumble it.
2. Add a pinch of salt and the onions to the same skillet with the bacon drippings, cooking until the onion is tender and lightly browned (around 3 minutes).
3. Then add water and mustard, stirring and scraping up any browned bits from the pan. Finally, add the Brussels sprouts and cook for 4-6 minutes, stirring occasionally, until they are tender.
4. Stir in a splash of vinegar and top with the crumbled bacon before serving.

Roasted Broccoli with Lemon, Garlic & Toasted Pine Nuts

INGREDIENTS
1 lb broccoli floret
2 tablespoons olive oil
salt & freshly ground black pepper
2 tablespoons unsalted butter
1 teaspoon garlic, minced
1/2 teaspoon lemon zest, grated
1 -2 tablespoon fresh lemon juice
2 tablespoons pine nuts, toasted

DIRECTIONS

1. Begin by preheating the oven to 500 degrees.
2. In a large bowl, mix the broccoli florets with some oil and season to taste with salt and pepper.
3. Spread the florets in a single layer on a baking sheet. Roast for 12 minutes, flipping halfway, until lightly cooked or just tender.
4. Melt the butter in a saucepan over medium heat.
5. Stir in the garlic and lemon zest and cook for one minute.
6. When done, take off the flame and combine with lemon juice.
7. Place the broccoli in a bowl, pour the lemon butter over it and mix together.
8. Sprinkle the toasted pine nuts over the top.

Vegan Lentil Burgers

INGREDIENTS

1 cup dry lentils, well rinsed

2 1/2 cups water

1/2 teaspoon salt

1 tablespoon olive oil

1/2 medium onion, diced

1 carrot, diced

1 teaspoon pepper

1 tablespoon soy sauce

3⁄4 cup rolled oats, finely ground
3⁄4 cup breadcrumbs

DIRECTIONS

1. Bring the lentils and salt to a boil in a pot of water, and allow them to cook for about 45 minutes. The lentils should be tender and most of the liquid should have evaporated.
2. Next, heat the oil in a skillet and add the onion and carrot. Cook it until it softens, and that should take only around 5 minutes.
3. Combine the cooked ingredients in a bowl with the pepper, soy sauce, oats, and bread crumbs until everything is mixed.
4. Once the mixture is still warm to the touch, shape it into patties. You should be able to make 8-10 burgers from this batch.
5. Finally, you can either shallow fry the burgers for 1-2 minutes on each side or bake them in an oven preheated to 200C for 15 minutes.

Sauerkraut Salad

INGREDIENTS
1 (1 lb) can sauerkraut, drained but not rinsed
1 cup celery, chopped fine
1⁄2 cup green pepper, chopped fine

2 tablespoons onions, chopped fine

1⁄2 teaspoon salt

1⁄2 teaspoon pepper

3⁄4 cup sugar

1⁄3 cup salad oil

1⁄3 cup cider (I use white) or 1/3 cup white vinegar (I use white)

DIRECTIONS

1. Chop up the vegetables and combine them with the sauerkraut.
2. Set a pot on low heat, and add sugar, oil, vinegar, salt, and pepper. Stir until the sugar melts completely.
3. Allow the mixture to cool off, then pour it over the vegetables.
4. Refrigerate overnight.

Sweet Potato Curry with Spinach and Chickpeas

INGREDIENTS

1⁄2 large sweet onions, chopped or 2 scallions, thinly sliced

1 -2 teaspoon canola oil

2 tablespoons curry powder

1 tablespoon cumin

1 teaspoon cinnamon

10 ounces fresh spinach, washed, stemmed and coarsely chopped

2 large sweet potatoes, peeled and diced (about 2 lbs)

1 (14 1/2 ounce) can chickpeas, rinsed and drained

1/2 cup water

1 (14 1/2 ounce) can diced tomatoes, can substitute fresh if available

1/4 cup chopped fresh cilantro, for garnish

basmati rice or brown rice, for serving

DIRECTIONS

1. The sweet potatoes can be cooked any way you like, but my favorite is peeling, chopping and steaming them in a veggie steamer for roughly fifteen minutes.
2. Baking and boiling are other options.
3. Now heat the 1-2 tsp of oil in a pan on medium heat, add the chopped onions and sauté for two to three minutes until softened.
4. Sprinkle in the curry powder, cumin, and cinnamon and stir to completely coat the onions.
5. Toss in the tomatoes with their liquid, plus the chickpeas and stir until blended.
6. Pour in half a cup of water and increase the heat to a strong simmer for one or two minutes.
7. Add handfuls of fresh spinach at a time, stirring it into the cooking liquid until all of it is incorporated.
8. Place the lid on to let it wilt for three minutes, then place in the cooked sweet potatoes and stir so they are covered in liquid.

9. Let the mixture simmer for three to five minutes, until all flavors are combined.
10. Serve on a platter and top with cilantro. This dish can be great served over basmati or brown rice.

Millet & Quinoa Mediterranean Salad

INGREDIENTS
1/2 cup millet
1 cup water
1/2 cup quinoa (red, white, or black)
3/4 cup water
1 English cucumber, diced
1 tomatoes, ripe, seeds squeezed out, diced
1 sweet pepper, seeded, diced
1/2 red onion, sliced thin
1 garlic clove, pressed
200 g feta cheese, diced
1 (10 ounce) can large white beans, drained
1/4 teaspoon cayenne pepper (more, to taste)
2 teaspoons dried dill (sub basil or oregano, if preferred)
1/4 cup pine nuts
1 lemon, juice of (zest as well, if preferred)
1 tablespoon olive oil (optional)
fresh ground pepper, to taste

DIRECTIONS

1. Pour the millet and 1 cup of water into a pot, and once it comes to a boil, reduce the heat and let it simmer for 5 minutes. Switch off the stove, cover it and let it rest for 10 minutes.
2. Pour the quinoa and ¾ of water into a pot and bring it to a boil. Once it is boiling reduce the heat and let it simmer covered for 12-14 minutes.
3. Mix and toss all the ingredients together and let it chill.

DINNER

Weeknight Chicken Wings

INGREDIENTS
1 pound (450 grams) raw, unbreaded chicken wings
seasoning blend or rub of your choice

DIRECTIONS

1. Preheat your oven to 360-395°F
2. Season the chicken with a spice of your and make sure to massage the spices in.
3. Place the seasoned chicken into the oven and back for about 40 minutes, or at least until all the wings are fully cooked.

4. To get the wings golden brown and crunchy, broil the wings flipping them occasionally. Make sure to man over the wings so they don't burn.
5. Serve with ranch dressing, and vegetables of your choice, can include celery and carrot sticks.

Supper Club Tilapia Parmesan

INGREDIENTS

2 lbs tilapia filets (orange roughy, cod or red snapper can be substituted)
2 tablespoons lemon juice
1/2 cup grated parmesan cheese
4 tablespoons butter, room temperature
3 tablespoons mayonnaise
3 tablespoons finely chopped green onions
1/4 teaspoon seasoning salt (I like Old Bay seasoning here)
1/4 teaspoon dried basil
black pepper
1 dash hot pepper sauce

DIRECTIONS

1. Preheat your oven to 350 degrees.
2. Arrange the filets in a single layer on a buttered 13-by-9-inch baking dish or jelly roll pan. Avoid stacking the filets.
3. Brush the top of the filets with juice.

4. In a bowl, mix cheese, butter, mayonnaise, onions, and seasonings with a fork until well combined.

5. Bake the fish in the preheated oven for 10 to 20 minutes, or until the fish starts to flake. Keep an eye on the fish to prevent overcooking.

6. Spread the cheese mixture over the fish and bake for an additional 5 minutes or until golden brown.

7. The baking time may vary depending on the thickness of the fish.

8. The recipe yields 4 servings.

9. Note: You can also make this fish in a broiler. Broil for 3 to 4 minutes or until almost done, then add cheese and broil for another 2 to 3 minutes or until browned.

Warm Roasted Vegetable Farro Salad

INGREDIENTS

1/2 medium sized eggplant, peel on and large diced

1 tablespoon kosher salt or 1 tablespoon sea salt

1 cup cherry tomatoes, washed and left whole

1 medium sized zucchini, peel on and large diced

6 white button mushrooms, quartered

6 garlic cloves, peeled, trimmed and sliced

1/2 medium sized red onion, peeled and cut into wedges

1 tablespoon olive oil

1 cup cracked farro

2 cups almond milk (Almond Breeze)

1 teaspoon tbsp olive oil (15 mL)

1 tablespoon olive oil

1 tablespoon balsamic vinegar

3 sprigs fresh cilantro

1/2 teaspoon salt

1/2 teaspoon pepper

DIRECTIONS

1. Preheat your oven to 400°F (200°C).
2. Salt the eggplant slices generously on all sides in a large flat pan or baking sheet, toss to coat evenly, and let them sit for 30 minutes to release excess moisture and bitterness. Drain and rinse the eggplant, then add it to a large mixing bowl with tomatoes, zucchini, mushrooms, garlic, and onions. Drizzle the vegetables generously with olive oil, season with salt and pepper, and stir to coat.
3. Transfer the vegetables to an ovenproof pan lined with tin foil and roast them in the preheated oven for 20-25 minutes or until they are soft, caramelized, and fork-tender. Stir or flip the vegetables 10-15 minutes into the roasting process to prevent them from sticking to the pan. Once done, remove the pan from the oven and set aside.
4. Meanwhile, rinse the farro with water and drain it in a colander over the sink. Add the farro to a 3-quart (3L) saucepot, pour in the Almond Breeze, and

season with a pinch of salt and a drizzle of olive oil. Bring the liquid to boil over medium-high heat, then reduce the heat to a low simmer to prevent spilling over. Simmer the farro for 20 minutes with the lid of the pot cocked to one side to let out steam. Once done, turn off the heat, leave the pot on the stovetop, and close the lid. Let the farro steam in the pot for another 5 minutes or until it is soft but slightly chewy in the center. Remove the lid and fluff the farro with a fork.

5. To assemble the dish, combine the cooked farro with the roasted vegetables in a large serving dish and gently toss to mix. Whisk together the olive oil with the balsamic vinegar and drizzle over the farro salad. Toss to coat and season with salt and pepper to taste. Garnish with fresh cilantro and a squeeze of lemon. Serve the dish warm.

Best Baked Potato

INGREDIENTS
1 large russet potato
canola oil
kosher salt

DIRECTIONS

1. Set the oven to 350°F and arrange the racks in the upper and lower thirds.
2. Thoroughly wash the potato (or potatoes) using a stiff brush and cold running water.
3. Dry the potato and use a standard fork to prick 8 to 12 deep holes all over it, allowing moisture to escape during cooking.
4. Coat the potato lightly with oil by placing it in a bowl and sprinkling it with kosher salt. Then, place the potato directly on the oven rack in the middle of the oven.
5. Place a baking sheet on the lower rack to catch any drippings during cooking.
6. Bake for 1 hour or until the skin feels crispy but the flesh underneath is soft.
7. To serve, use your fork to create a dotted line from end to end, and then crack the potato open by squeezing the ends towards each other. It should easily split open, but be careful because there will be some steam.
8. Note that if you are cooking more than 4 potatoes, you may need to extend the cooking time by up to 15 minutes.

Easy Black Bean Soup

INGREDIENTS

3 tablespoons olive oil

1 medium onion, chopped

1 tablespoon ground cumin

2 -3 cloves garlic

2 (14 1/2 ounce) cans black beans

2 cups chicken broth or 2 cups vegetable broth

salt and pepper

1 small red onion, chopped fine

1/4 cup cilantro, coarsely chopped or finely chopped (whatever you prefer)

DIRECTIONS

1. In a pot, sauté an onion in olive oil until it turns translucent.
2. Add cumin and cook for 30 seconds, then add garlic and continue cooking for another 30 to 60 seconds.
3. Pour in 1 can of black beans and 2 cups of vegetable broth, and bring the mixture to a simmer. Stir occasionally.
4. Turn off the heat, and using a hand blender, blend the ingredients in the pot. Alternatively, transfer the mixture to a blender and blend it.

5. Add the second can of black beans to the pot along with the blended ingredients, and bring it back to a simmer.

6. For garnish, serve the soup with bowls of red onion and cilantro. You can also add a bit of cilantro to the pot.

7. This recipe can be doubled or frozen.

Cajun Potato, Shrimp & Avocado Salad

INGREDIENTS

300g new potatoes (small baby or chats 10 oz halved)

1 tablespoon olive oil

250g king prawns (8 oz, cooked and peeled)

1 garlic clove (minced)

2 spring onions (finely sliced)

2 teaspoons cajun seasoning

1 avocado (peeled, stoned and diced)

1 cup alfalfa sprout

salt (to boil potatoes)

DIRECTIONS

1. In a large saucepan of lightly salted boiling water, cook the potatoes for 10 to 15 minutes or until tender. Drain well.

2. Heat oil in a wok or a large nonstick frying pan/skillet. Add prawns, garlic, spring onions, and

Cajun seasoning. Stir-fry for 2 to 3 minutes or until the prawns are hot.

3. Add the cooked potatoes to the wok or frying pan/skillet and cook for a further minute.
4. Transfer the mixture to serving dishes. Top with avocado and alfalfa sprouts before serving.

Baked Mahi Mahi

INGREDIENTS

2 lbs mahi mahi (4 filets)
1 lemon, juiced
1/4 teaspoon garlic salt
1/4 teaspoon ground black pepper
1 cup mayonnaise
1/4 cup white onion, finely chopped
breadcrumbs

DIRECTIONS

1. To prepare the baked fish, start by preheating the oven to 425°F. Then, rinse the fish and place it in a baking dish. Squeeze fresh lemon juice on the fish, followed by a sprinkle of garlic salt and pepper.
2. Next, mix mayonnaise and chopped onions in a bowl, then spread the mixture evenly over the fish. Finally, sprinkle bread crumbs over the top and bake the dish in the preheated oven for 25 minutes.

Broccoli Dal Curry

INGREDIENTS

4 tablespoons butter or 4 tablespoons ghee

2 medium onions, chopped

1 teaspoon chili powder

1 1/2 teaspoons black pepper

2 teaspoons cumin

1 teaspoon ground coriander

2 teaspoons turmeric

1 cup red lentil

1 lemon, juice of

3 cups chicken broth

2 medium broccoli, chopped

1/2 cup dried coconut (optional)

1 tablespoon flour

1 teaspoon salt

1 cup cashews, coarsely chopped (optional)

DIRECTIONS

1. Saute onions in butter in a saucepan until they are well-browned.
2. Sprinkle in the chili powder, cumin, coriander, pepper, and turmeric, and stir for 1 minute.
3. Add lentils, lemon juice, broth, and coconut (if desired).

4. Bring the mixture to a boil, then reduce the heat and simmer for 45-55 minutes. If the mixture is too thick, add some hot water.

5. Steam broccoli for 7 minutes, then immediately immerse in cold water and set aside.

6. Combine 1/3 cup of the lentil mixture's liquid from the simmering mixture with flour to create a smooth paste.

7. Return the paste to the pan, add broccoli, salt, and nuts (if using), and simmer for 5 minutes.

8. Serve with Basmati rice.

Sheet Pan Chicken & Brussels Sprouts

INGREDIENTS

4 skin on chicken thighs

1 1⁄2 cups Brussels sprouts, halved

4 carrots, cut on the bias

3 tablespoons olive oil

1 teaspoon herbes de provence

DIRECTIONS

1. Set the oven to 400° F to preheat.

2. Add 1½ tbsp olive oil, ½ tsp herbs, salt, and pepper to a bowl of cut vegetables. Rub the mixture all over the vegetables.

3. Put the vegetables on a sheet pan.

4. Place the chicken thighs in the same bowl. Drizzle with 1½ tbsp olive oil, ½ tsp herbs, salt, and pepper, then rub the mixture all over the chicken.

5. Place the chicken on the sheet pan with the vegetables.

6. Roast for approximately 30-35 minutes or until the chicken is fully cooked.

7. If you prefer crispier vegetables or chicken skin, turn on the broiler and cook for one or two minutes. Be careful not to let it burn, so watch it closely.

Perfect Cauliflower Pizza Crust

INGREDIENTS

4 cups raw cauliflower, riced or 1 medium cauliflower head

1 egg, beaten

1 1 cup chevre cheese or 1 cup other soft cheese

1 teaspoon dried oregano

1 pinch salt

DIRECTIONS

1. Initiate preheating of the oven to a temperature of 400°F.

2. For the preparation of cauliflower rice, grind batches of raw cauliflower florets in a food processor until they attain a texture similar to that of rice.

3. Proceed to fill a large pot with approximately an inch of water and bring it to a boiling point. Add the cauliflower "rice" and subsequently cover it. Allow it to cook for approximately 4-5 minutes. Drain the content into a fine-mesh strainer.

4. The secret step: Once the rice is drained, transfer it to a clean, thin dishtowel. Wrap the steamed rice in the dishtowel, twist it, and then drain all the extra moisture present. Astonishingly, a significant amount of additional liquid will be expelled, which will leave a desirable and dry pizza crust.

5. In a sizable bowl, mix the drained rice, beaten egg, goat cheese, and seasonings. Do not hesitate to use your hands as it is preferable to have a thoroughly mixed content. Although the resulting dough differs from conventional pizza dough, it will successfully stay together.

6. Subsequently, press the dough onto a baking sheet that is lined with parchment paper. It is imperative to use parchment paper to avoid the dough from sticking. Maintain the thickness of the dough to approximately 3/8" while making the edges slightly raised for a "crust" effect if desired.

7. Commence baking for approximately 35-40 minutes at 400°F. The crust should possess a firmness and a golden-brown hue when completed.

8. Now is the optimal moment to add your preferred toppings such as sauce, cheese, and any other desired

add-ons. Return the pizza to the 400°F oven and bake for an additional 5-10 minutes or until the cheese is melted and bubbling.

9. Finally, slice the pizza and serve it immediately.

Sweet Potato & Black Bean Burrito

INGREDIENTS

5 cups peeled cubed sweet potatoes

1/2 teaspoon salt

2 teaspoons other vegetable oil or 2 teaspoons broth

3 1/2 cups diced onions

4 garlic cloves, minced (or pressed)

1 tablespoon minced fresh green chili pepper

4 teaspoons ground cumin

4 teaspoons ground coriander

4 1/2 cups cooked black beans (three 15-ounce cans, drained)

2/3 cup lightly packed cilantro leaf

2 tablespoons fresh lemon juice

1 teaspoon salt

12 (10 inch) flour tortillas

fresh salsa

DIRECTIONS

1. Preheat the oven to 350 degrees Fahrenheit.
2. In a medium saucepan, combine the sweet potatoes, salt, and enough water to cover them.

3. Cover the saucepan and bring the mixture to a boil, then reduce heat and simmer for about 10 minutes until the sweet potatoes are tender.

4. Drain the sweet potatoes and set them aside.

5. Meanwhile, heat the oil in a medium skillet over medium-low heat.

6. Add the onions, garlic, and chile to the skillet and cover it.

7. Cook the vegetables, stirring occasionally, until the onions are tender (about 7 minutes).

8. Add the cumin and coriander to the skillet and cook, stirring frequently, for 2 to 3 minutes longer.

9. Remove the skillet from heat and set it aside.

10. In a food processor, combine the black beans, cilantro, lemon juice, salt, and cooked sweet potatoes and blend until smooth (or mash the ingredients in a large bowl by hand).

11. Transfer the sweet potato mixture to a large mixing bowl and mix in the cooked onions and spices.

12. Lightly oil a large baking dish.

13. Spoon about 2/3 to 3/4 cup of the filling in the center of each tortilla, roll it up, and place it seam-side down in the baking dish.

14. Cover the dish tightly with foil and bake it for about 30 minutes or until piping hot.

15. Serve the enchiladas topped with salsa.

Slow Cooker Black-Eyed Peas

INGREDIENTS

1 (16 ounce) bag dried black-eyed peas

1 small ham hock

1 (14 1/2 ounce) can Del Monte zesty jalapeno pepper diced tomato

1 (14 1/2 ounce) can diced tomatoes with green chilies

2 (10 1/2 ounce) cans chicken broth

1 stalk celery, chopped

DIRECTIONS

1. Follow the soaking instructions of the black-eyed peas as specified on the packaging.
2. Mix all the ingredients and slow cook for 9-10 on low heat.

Meatza

INGREDIENTS

1/2 pound (225 grams) ground Italian sausage

1/4 cup (60 grams) pizza sauce

1/3 cup (40 grams) shredded pizza cheese

your preferred pizza toppings

DIRECTIONS

1. Preheat the oven to 375°F (190°C).
2. Start by forming the sausage into a thin layer on a nonstick rimmed baking sheet. Bake it in the oven until fully cooked, then drain away any extra grease.
3. Cover the sausage with sauce, cheese, and toppings.
4. Put the baking sheet back in the oven and let the cheese melt and brown, which should take 10–15 minutes.

Shortcut Fajitas

INGREDIENTS
1 tablespoon (15 mL) coconut oil
1 red onion, sliced
2 bell peppers, sliced
1 1/2 cups (210 grams) shredded cooked chicken (from a rotisserie chicken, if available)
fajita seasoning, salt, and pepper
water, as needed
lettuce
tomato

FAJITA SEASONING:

Combine chili, garlic and onion powder to create your own fajita seasoning.

DIRECTIONS

1. Heat up a large skillet with oil on medium-high heat.
2. Pour in the onion and bell peppers and saute until the vegetables begin to turn brown. Just ensure they are still crispy.
3. Add the chicken, sprinkling in the seasonings and add 1-2 tablespoons of water if needed to help the veggies and meat absorb the seasoning.
4. Cook the chicken until it is done, or to your liking and remove it from the heat.
5. Serve the chicken on some low carb tortillas with some lettuce, tomato and sour cream, Enjoy!

Low-Carb Chicken Nuggets

INGREDIENTS

1 egg, beaten
1/2 cup (48 grams) almond flour
1/2 cup (45 grams) grated Parmesan cheese
salt and pepper
1 boneless, skinless chicken breast, cut into nugget-size pieces
olive oil cooking spray

DIRECTIONS

1. In a medium-sized bowl, crack and beat an egg well.
2. In another bowl add the almond flour , parmesan, salt and pepper and mix it well.
3. Place the chicken pieces in the egg bowl first. Remember to not overcrowd as you want all your pieces properly coated in egg, then roll the egged pieces in the almond mixture bowl until the whole piece is coated.
4. Spray an airfryer basket with cooking spray, then add the breaded pieces into the basket. Spray the nuggets with cooking spray as this will help them retain the golden brown hue.
5. Cook the nuggets at 373°F (190°C) for 5 minutes, then flip the nuggets and cook them further for another 5 minutes.
6. You can serve the nuggets with a low carb dipping sauce of your choice and a nice side salad.

Cauliflower Rice Taco Bowls

INGREDIENTS
cauliflower rice
cooked, taco-seasoned ground beef
red onion
lime wedges
shredded cheese

sour cream

cilantro

guacamole

salsa

lettuce

radish slices

taco sauce

DIRECTIONS

1. Nicely lay out all the ingredients in a sharing or self-service-style.
2. Everyone can prepare their own bowl as they like.

Easy Zucchini Spaghetti

INGREDIENTS

1 pound (450 grams) lean ground beef

salt

4 medium zucchini, spiralized

1 (24-ounce / 700-mL) jar no-sugar-added spaghetti sauce

grated Parmesan cheese

DIRECTIONS

1. In a skillet on medium heat, cook the beef till it's done.

2. At the same time, salt the zucchini noodles to get rid of any moisture.

3. Afterwards, eliminate any fat remaining from the beef.

4. Turn down the heat, add the sauce and the noodles to the pan. Let it heat through.

5. When it's time to serve, sprinkle each portion with Parmesan cheese.

7-DAY MEAL PLANS

Below are four meal plans to get you started, but at this point I need to stress a couple of things. The first is that while the times run from 10am to 5pm in the left-hand column, obviously if your window is 12pm to 8pm then disregard the times shown. The second thing is to feel free to substitute any of the suggestions for ones that you'd prefer. All the recipes mentioned are laid out in detail above. But maybe you don't like tofu, or maybe you don't have the ingredients at home to make the suggested choice. All they are is suggestions, but by all means do your own thing if you'd prefer. One way to do this is to look at the Table of Contents of this book each day and pick a breakfast, snack, lunch and dinner from the list that you feel like and that you have the ingredients for (obviously shopping in advance would avoid that scenario). And if you don't mind having the same thing twice or more each week, then make a big batch, saving you time and washing-up!

The last thing to note is that I've assumed dinner will take about an hour, so for example in Meal Plan 1 breakfast is at 10am and dinner is 7 hours later at 5pm, because I'm assuming you'll finish around 6pm, so your eating window is therefore 10am-6pm, i.e. 8 hours.

Meal Plan 1

Day 1:

Time	Meal
10 am breakfast:	French Vanilla Almond Granola
11 am snack:	Trail Mix
2 pm lunch:	Avocado Waldorf Chicken Salad
5 pm dinner:	Broccoli Dal Curry

Day 2:

Time	Meal
10 am breakfast:	Summer Berry Crisp
1 pm lunch:	Bunless Butter Burger
3 pm snack:	Cauliflower Popcorn
5 pm dinner:	Weeknight Chicken Wings

Day 3:

Time	Meal
10 am breakfast:	Peach Berry Smoothie
11 am snack:	Spicy Chocolate Keto Fat Bombs
1 pm lunch:	Grilled Lemon Salmon
5 pm dinner:	Supper Club Tilapia Parmesan

Day 4:

Time	Meal
10 am breakfast:	Poached Eggs and Avocado Toast
11 am snack:	Cauliflower Popcorn
2 pm lunch:	Cobb Salad with Brown Derby Dressing
5 pm dinner:	Easy Black Bean Soup

Day 5:

Time	Meal
10 am breakfast:	The Easiest Hard-Boiled Eggs
1 pm lunch:	Vegan Fried 'Fish' Tacos
3 pm snack:	Trail Mix
5 pm dinner:	Cajun Potato, Shrimp & Avocado Salad

Day 6:

Time	Meal
10 am breakfast:	Avocado Quesadillas
11 am snack:	Vegan Coconut Kefir Banana Muffins
2 pm lunch:	Mediterranean Chicken Breasts with Avocado Tapenade
5 pm dinner:	Baked Mahi Mahi

Day 7:

Time	Meal
10 am breakfast:	Egg and Veggie Scramble
1 pm lunch:	Shredded Brussel Sprouts with Bacon & Onions
3 pm snack:	Cauliflower Popcorn
5 pm dinner:	Sweet Potato & Black Bean Burrito

Meal Plan 2

The second meal plan is similar to the first, but the eating window has changed and so has the order of the types of meal. Feel free to change the order and the timings to suit your life.

Day 1:

Time	Meal
11 am breakfast:	Overnight Chia Pudding
2 pm lunch:	Millet & Quinoa Mediterranean Salad
4 pm snack:	Cheese Bites
6 pm dinner:	Easy Zucchini Spaghetti

Day 2:

Time	Meal
11 am breakfast:	Bacon and Eggs
2 pm lunch:	Sweet Potato Curry with Spinach and Chickpeas
4 pm snack:	Smoked Salmon Spread
6 pm dinner:	Cauliflower Rice Taco Bowls

Day 3:

Time	Meal
11 am breakfast:	Avocado Quesadillas
2 pm lunch:	Sauerkraut Salad
4 pm snack:	Bacon-Wrapped Scallops
6 pm dinner:	Low-Carb Chicken Nuggets

Day 4:

Time	Meal
11 am breakfast:	The Easiest Hard-Boiled Eggs
2 pm lunch:	Vegan Lentil Burgers
4 pm snack:	Toasted Ravioli
6 pm dinner:	Shortcut Fajitas

Day 5:

Time	Meal
11 am breakfast:	French Vanilla Almond Granola
2 pm lunch:	Mediterranean Chicken Breasts with Avocado Tapenade
4 pm snack:	Zucchini Bites
6 pm dinner:	Meatza

Day 6:

Time	Meal
11 am breakfast:	Poached Eggs and Avocado Toast
2 pm lunch:	Veggie-Packed Cheesy Chicken Salad
4 pm snack:	Hot and Spicy Peanuts
6 pm dinner:	Slow Cooker Black-Eyed Peas

Day 7:

Time	Meal
11 am breakfast:	Egg and Veggie Scramble
2 pm lunch:	Grilled Lemon Salmon
4 pm snack:	Trail Mix
6 pm dinner:	Perfect Cauliflower Pizza Crust

Meal Plan 3

Another variation for you.

Day 1:

Time	Meal
12 pm breakfast:	Summer Berry Crisp
2 pm snack:	Spicy Chocolate Keto Fat Bombs
3 pm lunch:	Bunless Butter Burger
7 pm dinner:	Weeknight Chicken Wings

Day 2:

Time	Meal
12 pm breakfast:	Peach Berry Smoothie
2 pm snack:	Cauliflower Popcorn
3 pm lunch:	Grilled Lemon Salmon
7 pm dinner:	Supper Club Tilapia Parmesan

Day 3:

Time	Meal
12 pm breakfast:	French Vanilla Almond Granola
2 pm snack:	Vegan Coconut Kefir Banana Muffins
3 pm lunch:	Avocado Waldorf Chicken Salad
7 pm dinner:	Warm Roasted Vegetable Farro Salad

Day 4:

Time	Meal
12 pm breakfast:	Poached Eggs and Avocado Toast
2 pm snack:	Trail Mix
3 pm lunch:	Veggie-Packed Cheesy Chicken Salad
7 pm dinner:	Best Baked Potato

Day 5:

Time	Meal
12 pm breakfast:	The Easiest Hard-boiled Eggs
2 pm snack:	Caramelized Onion-Cranberry Cream Cheese Bites
3 pm lunch:	Cobb Salad with Brown Derby Dressing
7 pm dinner:	Easy Black Bean Soup

Day 6:

Time	Meal
12 pm breakfast:	Avocado Quesadillas
2 pm snack:	Pizza Meatloaf Cups
3 pm lunch:	Vegan Fried 'Fish' Tacos
7 pm dinner:	Cajun Potato, Shrimp & Avocado Salad

Day 7:

Time	Meal
12 pm breakfast:	Egg and Veggie Scramble
2 pm snack:	Cheese Bites
3 pm lunch:	Mediterranean Chicken Breasts with Avocado Tapenade
7 pm dinner:	Baked Mahi Mahi

Meal Plan 4

The last one shifts the time back an hour, but again if you prefer different timings just use the meal suggestions and disregard the timings.

Day 1:

Time	Meal
11 am breakfast:	Bacon and Eggs
2 pm lunch:	Shredded Brussels Sprouts with Bacon & Onions
4 pm snack:	Smoked Salmon Spread
6 pm dinner:	Broccoli Dal Curry

Day 2:

Time	Meal
11 am breakfast:	Overnight Chia Pudding
2 pm lunch:	Roasted Broccoli with Lemon, Garlic & Toasted Pine Nuts
4 pm snack:	Bacon-Wrapped Scallops
6 pm dinner:	Sheet Pan Chicken & Brussels Sprouts

Day 3:

Time	Meal
11 am breakfast:	Summer Berry Crisp
2 pm lunch:	Vegan Lentil Burgers
4 pm snack:	Toasted Ravioli
6 pm dinner:	Perfect Cauliflower Pizza Crust

Day 4:

Time	Meal
11 am breakfast:	Poached Eggs and Avocado Toast
2 pm lunch:	Sauerkraut Salad
4 pm snack:	Zucchini Bites
6 pm dinner:	Sweet Potato & Black Bean Burrito

Day 5:

Time	Meal
11 am breakfast:	Egg and Veggie Scramble
2 pm lunch:	Sweet Potato Curry with Spinach and Chickpeas
4 pm snack:	Hot and Spicy Peanuts
6 pm dinner:	Slow Cooker Black-Eyed Peas

Day 6:

Time	Meal
11 am breakfast:	Peach Berry Smoothie
2 pm lunch:	Millet & Quinoa Mediterranean Salad
4 pm snack:	Cauliflower Popcorn
6 pm dinner:	Meatza

Day 7:

Time	Meal
11 am breakfast:	French Vanilla Almond Granola
2 pm lunch:	Mediterranean Chicken Breasts with Avocado Tapenade
4 pm snack:	Bacon-Wrapped Scallops
6 pm dinner:	Low-Carb Chicken Nuggets

CONCLUSION

I'm glad you've made it this far. It should tell you that you're serious about going on this journey, which means that you're going to succeed. Let's just finish up with a recap. In no particular order:

Try and start with 16:8 to give yourself the best chance of success.

Move up to it in stages from your current fasting:eating window, to make the transition as easy as possible.

Try and start when the plan for your week is known so that you can avoid unplanned meals.

Don't be hard on yourself. Allow yourself a day off every now and then. This is a marathon not a sprint.

Remind yourself why you're doing it, often.

Please be patient. Results will come.

Weigh yourself if you can.

Join Facebook groups for motivation. Having people who are going through the same thing really helps.

Throw in a longer fast now and then.

If you do all that, in a few weeks you'll be wondering why you didn't try this years ago. Go for it! Good luck! You've got this!

PASSING THE BATON

I hope you feel that this book delivered what it promised, namely to equip you with the knowledge and techniques to finally get the results you are looking for in terms of weight, energy and outlook.

Simply by leaving your honest opinion of this book on Amazon, you'll show other women who are starting out on the same journey where they can find the information they're looking for.

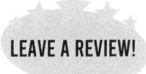

LEAVE A REVIEW!

Thank you for your help. This way of life is kept alive when we pass on our knowledge – and you're helping me to do just that.

Scan the QR code to leave a review!

REFERENCES

1 Hall, K. D. (2018, January 1). *Maintenance of lost weight and long-term management of obesity*. NIH - Library of Medicine. https://www.ncbi.nlm.nih.gov/pmc/articles/PMC5764193/
tinyurl.com/weightif

2 Edwards, M. (2022, July 18). *Biochemistry, Lipolysis*. National Library of Medicine. https://www.ncbi.nlm.nih.gov/books/NBK560564/
tinyurl.com/fastlipo

3 Anton, S. (2018, February 1). *Flipping the Metabolic Switch: Understanding and Applying Health Benefits of Fasting*. National Library of Medicine. https://www.ncbi.nlm.nih.gov/pmc/articles/PMC5783752/
tinyurl.com/flipif

4 Qian, J. (2021, October 1). *Innate immune remodeling by short-term intensive fasting*. National Library of Medicine. https://www.ncbi.nlm.nih.gov/pmc/articles/PMC8590100/
tinyurl.com/autofast

5 The Journal of Clinical Endocrinology & Metabolism (1992, April 1). *Augmented growth hormone (GH) secretory burst frequency and amplitude mediate enhanced GH secretion during a two-day fast in normal men*. JCEM. https://academic.oup.com/jcem/article-abstract/74/4/757/3004645?redirectedFrom=fulltext
tinyurl.com/ghfast

6 National Institutes of Health (2014, June 5). *Prolonged fasting reduces IGF-1/PKA to promote hematopoietic-stem-cell-based regeneration and reverse immunosuppression*. National Library of Medicine. https://pubmed.ncbi.nlm.nih.gov/24905167/
tinyurl.com/regenfast

7 Bagherniya, M. (2018, October 1). *The effect of fasting or calorie restriction on autophagy induction: A review of the literature*. PubMed. https://pubmed.ncbi.nlm.nih.gov/30172870/
tinyurl.com/moreauto

8 National Institutes of Health (2022, March 24). Effect of Intermittent

Fasting Diet on Glucose and Lipid Metabolism and Insulin Resistance in Patients with Impaired Glucose and Lipid Metabolism: A Systematic Review and Meta-Analysis. National Library of Medicine. https://www.ncbi.nlm.nih.gov/pmc/articles/PMC8970877/
tinyurl.com/insulinif

9 National Institutes of Health (2020, October 1). *Fasting Drives Nrf2-Related Antioxidant Response in Skeletal Muscle.* National Library of Medicine. https://www.ncbi.nlm.nih.gov/pmc/articles/PMC7589317/
tinyurl.com/antioxif

10 National Institutes of Health (2005, March 1). *Beneficial effects of intermittent fasting and caloric restriction on the cardiovascular and cerebrovascular systems.* National Library of Medicine. https://pubmed.ncbi.nlm.nih.gov/15741046/
tinyurl.com/cardioif

11 National Institutes of Health (2016, July 11). *Fasting mimicking diet reduces HO-1 to promote T cell-mediated tumor cytotoxicity.* National Library of Medicine. https://www.ncbi.nlm.nih.gov/pmc/articles/PMC5388544/
tinyurl.com/chemofast

12 National Institutes of Health (2019, May 1). *Intermittent Fasting: A Promising Approach for Preventing Vascular Dementia.* National Library of Medicine. https://www.ncbi.nlm.nih.gov/pmc/articles/PMC7379085/
tinyurl.com/dementiaif

13 Harvard School of Public Health (n.d.). *Diet Review: Intermittent Fasting for Weight Loss.* The Nutrition Source. https://www.hsph.harvard.edu/nutritionsource/healthy-weight/diet-reviews/intermittent-fasting/
tinyurl.com/harvardifreview

14 National Institutes of Health (2020, January 1). *Menopause-Associated Lipid Metabolic Disorders and Foods Beneficial for Postmenopausal Women.* National Library of Medicine. https://www.ncbi.nlm.nih.gov/pmc/articles/PMC7019719/
tinyurl.com/lipidif

15 National Institutes of Health (2019, June 1). *Aging of the Musculoskeletal System: How the Loss of Estrogen Impacts Muscle Strength.* National Library of Medicine. https://www.ncbi.nlm.nih.gov/pmc/articles/PMC6491229/
tinyurl.com/muscleif

16 National Institutes of Health (2012, December 1). *Analysis of the Degree of*

Insulin Resistance in Post Menopausal Women by Using Skin Temperature Measurements and Fasting Insulin and Fasting Glucose Levels: A Case Control Study. National Library of Medicine. https://www.ncbi.nlm.nih.gov/pmc/articles/PMC3552195

tinyurl.com/insulinif2

Made in the USA
Coppell, TX
29 April 2024

31858965R00089